Creating Myself

Creating Myself

How I Learned That Beauty Comes in All Shapes, Sizes, and Packages, Including Me

Mia Tyler

ATRIA BOOKS

New York   London   Toronto   Sydney

ATRIA BOOKS
A Division of Simon & Schuster, Inc.
1230 Avenue of the Americas
New York, NY 10020

First Atria Books hardcover edition June 2008

ATRIA BOOKS and colophon are trademarks of Simon & Schuster, Inc.

For information about special discounts for bulk purchases,
please contact Simon & Schuster Special Sales at
1-800-456-6798 or business@simonandschuster.com.

Designed by Nancy Singer

All photos courtesy of the author except as noted.

Manufactured in the United States of America

10 9 8 7 6 5 4 3 2 1

Library of Congress Cataloging-in-Publication Data

Tyler, Mia.
    Creating myself : how I learned that beauty comes in all shapes, sizes, and
packages, including me / by Mia Tyler.—1st Atria Books hardcover ed.
        p.   cm.
    Includes bibliographical references.
    1. Tyler, Mia.   2. Models (Persons)—Biography.   3. Children of
celebrities—Biography.   I. Title.

    HD8039.M77T95   A3   2008
    746.9'2092—dc22
    [B]   2008014121

ISBN-13: 978-1-4165-5860-6
ISBN-10:   1-4165-5860-8

This book is dedicated to you . . . May the journey of my life help you in creating your own story.

I just want everyone to stop judging others, stop hating, and realize we are all beautiful in our own ways. We shouldn't have to answer to anyone who thinks otherwise. Therefore we mustn't all be the same kind of person. I want everyone to just be themselves and tell anyone who says otherwise to screw off.

Everything in this book is true to the best of my ability to recall events. I have changed some names. I have also altered the names in and the content of the e-mails referred to and quoted in the text in order to protect the privacy of individuals who have corresponded with me on sensitive issues. But their messages have remained true. I treasure all the trust people have put in me.

Wanting to be someone else is a waste of the person you are.

—Kurt Cobain

Every life has a measure of sorrow, and sometimes this is what awakens us.

—Steven Tyler

I think I'm constantly in a state of adjustment.

—Patti Smith

As usual, there is a great woman behind every idiot.

—John Lennon

Sex kittens don't get fat. They get fluffy.

—Cyrinda Foxe

_____

[write your own quote]   —You

Contents

Prologue: The End   1

PART ONE

One   Liner Notes   9

Two   A New York Doll   14

Three   Walk This Way   18

Four   What Do You Do with a Baby   21

Five   There Is No Santa   27

Six   Night Terrors   33

Seven   Naked Nuns and the Bad Seed   39

Eight   The Facts of Life   45

Nine   The Problem with Cars   50

Ten   Sisters   54

Eleven   The Day the Roof Caved In   63

            A Good Place Inside Me   67

Contents

PART TWO

Twelve	The Urban Symphony	73
Thirteen	Fat Camp	79
Fourteen	Learning My Part	86
Fifteen	This Is the Life	90
Sixteen	Damn, Still Here	97
Seventeen	What Drugs Do You Have?	103
Eighteen	Sweet 16	109
Nineteen	A Scary Sight	116
Twenty	Dream On	121
	Don't Want the Pain	**127**

PART THREE

Twenty-one	Red Marks	133
Twenty-two	City Ass	139
Twenty-three	Help, I'm Going Crazy	147
Twenty-four	Promises	152
Twenty-five	V-Girl	159
Twenty-six	I'm Not a Model	164
Twenty-seven	Plus-sized	169
Twenty-eight	My Time in the Sun	176
Twenty-nine	Fan Mail	185
	MySpace	**191**

PART FOUR

Thirty	A New Boyfriend	197
Thirty-one	Cancer	205

Thirty-two	Amends	213
Thirty-three	Matching Stars	219
Thirty-four	Just Kissing	225
Thirty-five	Lesson Learned	231
Thirty-six	The M-Word	238
Thirty-seven	I Do, I Do, I *Think* I Do	244
Thirty-eight	Careful What You Wish For	250
Thirty-nine	Going Solo	257

A Reason, a Season, or a Lifetime **261**

PART FIVE

Forty	Starting Over	265
Forty-one	A Premonition	273
Forty-two	Good Looking Out	280

Acknowledgments 287

The End

On a warm spring night in 2001, a few months before my twenty-second birthday, I had an absurdly stupid, pathetic, and desperate thought—one few would have suspected coming from me, a successful plus-sized model featured in magazines and typically described as a self-confident role model.

I was going to kill myself.

I was up in the Hollywood Hills, at a home filled with a couple dozen people partying their brains out, some jumping naked in the pool and others dancing to music that thumped loud enough to feel like a series of small earthquakes.

Was it possible to be around so many people and still feel absolutely alone? Yes, sadly, and I was proof.

I opened a sliding door and stepped out onto a balcony that was cantilevered over a deep canyon. Standing there, I had the sense of being on a platform over nothing, a six-foot-long sidewalk suspended in the sky. Straight ahead, far beyond the drop, in a carpet of twinkling lights, clouds, and stars, sprawled Los Angeles, the City of Angels. Corny as it sounds, I wondered where my angels were, whether they were out there, and if they were, would I find them?

One thing I knew for sure. If I jumped, no one would find me at the bottom of the canyon.

I sat down and let my legs dangle over the edge. I puffed on a joint that I'd brought out with me and tried to figure out how I'd ended up in this spot—me, the daughter of rock star Steven Tyler and legendary '70s glamour girl Cyrinda Foxe. I knew better than to think that a gold American Express card and a famous last name guaranteed anything more in life than entry to a club. Then, as in the past, I had to ask if I wanted to be anyplace where they only cared about my last name.

What about me? What about my first name?

But never mind how other people reacted to me and what they thought. What did I think? How did I feel about me?

Why was it worthwhile going on? Was I happy? Had I ever been happy? Was there any meaning to my life?

Those questions and others went through my head. After I found myself repeating the word *no,* as in no, I'd never been happy, and no, there wasn't any meaning to my life, I stood up, gripped the rail with both hands, and with tears streaming from my eyes I prepared to jump.

Thoughts of the past and the future vanished from my head as I girded myself for whatever the end would feel like and the start of the next experience, if there was indeed some kind of life after death. I felt my heart beating fast and hard, and I filled up with fear. I wondered if it was going to hurt. If it did, it wouldn't matter for more than an instant, right?

Then, as I began to count my breaths toward the last one, I looked up at the sky. Through puddled eyes, I searched the stars and, though not religious, I asked God for a reason not to jump.

"Just give me a sign," I cried softly. "God, please give me a sign if I'm supposed to go on. I don't care what it is. Just give me something that will let me feel like I have a reason to face tomorrow."

Nothing happened.

"God?"

I don't know why, but I was waiting.

Less than ten seconds later, my cell phone rang. The sound

startled me. I didn't get service up in the hills. I took my phone out of my pocket anyway and saw that I had a message. I noticed that it had come in earlier that day, but due to what I supposed was bad cell reception, it didn't get to me until that moment.

What a moment, though. Right?

The message was from a talent executive at MTV saying that I'd been hired as the network's new metal chick VJ. He wanted me to return to New York immediately.

"We know you don't have any experience doing this," he said. "But we saw your tape and we like who you are. So let me know when you can get back here and we'll get you on air."

I listened to the message again. Then I sat down cross-legged on the balcony and cried till I ran out of energy.

Knowing that call had saved my life, I was overwhelmed by emotion. More important than the job was the message itself. Someone had found something worthwhile about me when I had no sense of my own self-worth. Someone wanted me when I was ready to give up. The timing was freakishly amazing. I'd asked for a sign and received a clear statement.

We like you.

That moment was a point when my life seemed to stop and restart, like rebooting a computer after it freezes. Some of the reasons for that were immediately obvious (like the fact that I didn't kill myself) and others became clear to me as I worked to figure out why I didn't like myself, why I was so unhappy, what I was supposed to do with my life, and how I could change to make things better. I remember saying to myself, "One day the pain will be worth it."

At various times I could only hope that was true—and fortunately it's worked out. Transformation is a lifelong process. The sun doesn't come out overnight. It didn't for me—and I still have days when the sky is dark and gloomy. But you can change no matter how desperate or dire your circumstances are. For me, it began with baby steps in a direction other than the one I'd been going. In other words, I faced my demons instead of running from them. That was never more true than when my mother lost her eighteen-month battle with brain cancer in 2002, and that's what this book is really about: dealing with life rather than hiding from it.

When I was three years old, Aerosmith guitarist Joe Perry's wife gave me a big brown-and-white quilt. It was uglier than sin, and I loved it. I wrapped myself in it, wore it like a queen's cape, and if anything shitty happened, which it inevitably did, I hid beneath it. I felt safe under it. It was my secret place, my safe haven.

In writing this book, I want to talk about the things that made me hide under that blanket, and more importantly, I want to talk about the changes I went through when I finally came out from under it. My hope is that one day someone will pick up this book, recognize themselves in these pages, and find hope, strength, and some direction from the way I dealt with my problems. If nothing else, they'll know they aren't alone—something I frequently wished I'd felt as I struggled through difficult times.

I receive thousands of e-mails every week from people wanting help or advice as they deal with issues that are too familiar to me: body image, drug abuse and alcoholism, cutting, sexual abuse, and simply feeling fucked up and cast off. Recently, a seventeen-year-old girl wrote to me about feeling unloved and neglected by her father. "I've drank myself to the point where I can't feel anything," she wrote. "I've cut myself to the point of passing out. I've smoked pot, snorted pills, and slept with and dated and thought I fell in love with too many different guys just because I needed someone to say they were here for me, cared about me, and noticed when I was not okay."

Another girl corresponded about her suicidal thoughts. "Today I thought I'd lost the battle and thought life would be better without me."

Do I know all the answers? No, and I don't pretend to know them. At twenty-eight, I'm still asking the questions. With my black hair and tattoos, I may look like I have a little more edge than most people, but inside I'm pretty normal. I freak out when I lose my ATM card. I'm addicted to handbags. I just paid a huge bill to the vet. I wish I had more money. Last week was just shitty, but a few weeks before that I got engaged and talked seriously about having babies. In other words, I'm living every day just like everyone else. Sometimes it's good. Other times it sucks.

Life doesn't happen by itself. There's no magic formula. There's no book of directions to follow. There's no map leading to the place you want to end up. A situation that seems overwhelming is really part of an ocean of experiences. You have to push through. Keep on truckin', as the saying goes. Don't stay in a rut. Don't look to blame other people. Look for solutions.

If there's a reason I'm around today to write this book, it's because I discovered a powerful message in a simple phrase. I think it was coined by motivator Scott Ginsberg, but I first came across it elsewhere.

Anyway, it's this: Life isn't about finding yourself. It's about creating yourself. I think that's a message to wake up to every day.

And as you'll see, I'm a work in progress—and that's a good thing.

Part One

Now and then when I see her face

She takes me away to that special place

—*Guns N' Roses*
"Sweet Child O'Mine"

ONE

Liner Notes

My dad's offhand comment caught me by surprise. We were on our way to New Hampshire to see his parents. We had started our road trip in Massachusetts, where my dad lived. Dad was behind the wheel, while I enjoyed the view from the passenger seat, realizing how much I liked the lush countryside and dense woods compared to the concrete and crowds of New York City, where I lived.

This was the first time Dad and I had ever been alone for this length of time, and it gave us time to talk without interruption, a rarity around him.

We caught each other up on our recent travels and personal lives, then lapsed easily into conversation about the past. For us, it was always a favorite topic. In our own ways, both of us were interested in figuring out what the hell had happened back then. The past was also a fitting topic since we were going to spend the night at the family home on the lake in Sunapee, where I grew up.

"By the way, you should go over to the Gray House and see if you want any of the stuff in it," he said. "I'm going to tear it down."

Wow. The Gray House was an old four-bedroom home. It was

next door to the larger, nicer, and completely refurbished residence where I had lived until I turned eleven. I shut my eyes and pictured both places perfectly. Images of my mom and me flooded my head. I could even see the power cords that my mom had run across the lawn from the big home into the Gray House after circumstances had forced us into the less desirable place. We'd stayed there for a year before moving to New York.

"What's in there?" I asked.

"I don't know," my dad said. "You gotta look around."

I could only imagine. Our move to the city had been abrupt and hurried, like an escape, even though there was nothing to escape at the time other than my mom's inability to restart her life after splitting from my dad. Our stuff must've still been in the Gray House sixteen years after we'd left it.

"Take anything you don't want thrown out," he added. "It's probably a bunch of junk."

"Hey," I said, pretending to take offense, "are you calling my New Kids on the Block posters junk?"

The conversation moved on to my mom. On a very personal level, one of the benefits of my dad's fame is that he has given so many interviews that few subjects are off-limits in conversation. He will, and can, talk about anything, including my mom. She was a sore, confusing, frustrating, and sad subject for both of us. My dad had divorced her, and I'd never liked her. Scratch that. I was angry at her for being so unhappy and not doing anything about it. When she died from brain cancer in 2002, I was relieved to know that she no longer had to suffer, but goddamn it, I was pissed at her for having wasted so much time being miserable and feeling sorry for herself.

"I should've tried to get her into rehab when I went," he said of the time he got sober in the late '80s. "Maybe things would've been different."

"Maybe," I said. "But you don't know if they'd have been better or worse."

"But your mom—"

I shushed him.

"I'd be a different person, not who I am today," I said. "And I like the way I've turned out. Mommy lived her life a certain way. You did, too. No regrets."

As soon as my dad turned down the dirt road leading to the house, I craned my head from side to side, trying to see everything at once. Suddenly there weren't enough windows in the car. I hadn't been back for a while, yet the familiarity of this place that I still considered home rushed at me until I was swamped by memories that hung in my brain like mental sticky notes.

The main house looked the same from the outside, but the interior had been redone by my stepmother in a faux Native American theme that made me think of cheap hotels and tacky souvenir shops. I didn't mention anything to my dad. After dinner, I spent the night in my old room and had weird dreams about my mom that disappeared as soon as I opened my eyes.

The next day, following a warm visit with my grandparents, I walked around the property. I wanted to take in the smells and feel of the woods and the lake. If New York was on one side of the planet, this felt like the opposite end. I was in no hurry to get to the Gray House, and when I finally did walk up to the front door I was telling myself that it wasn't a big deal.

I was wrong. As soon as I opened the front door, which was unlocked, I felt as if I had stepped into a time warp. It was a sci-fi movie starring me in dual roles, as myself in the present and as a little girl in the past. Weird. For a moment, I expected to see my mom come around the corner and tell me that I was going to lose my TV if I didn't clean my room. I shook my head. I could almost see myself unplugging the TV in my room and putting it in the hall outside my bedroom door.

That made me laugh. I so didn't give a shit about being in trouble as a kid.

Then I blinked a few times and returned to the present. I walked through several of the downstairs rooms until I came to a few large, green, extra-strength garbage bags. I knew they held the stuff I probably cared about, all of it crammed together and sealed with a twisted tie like time capsules.

One by one, I opened the bags and rummaged through them. I actually found myself having fun. Why hadn't I studied archaeology in school? Better question: why hadn't I studied, period? At any rate, I wasn't expecting to find anything of value or interest, but I surprised myself when I found a couple of my old sketchbooks. I sat down and looked through them. The pages were filled with drawings (horses and landscapes) and poems (variations on the "I hate my mother" theme). They came back to me as if I'd just done them.

From another bag, I pulled out some costume jewelry. I also found a couple books that meant something to me. Ah yes, then I came upon my old posters of Axl Rose, Sebastian Bach, and the New Kids on the Block, who were as cute as when I'd last seen them on my bedroom wall.

I spent a couple hours sifting through things, and at the end of that time I sat in the midst of a pile of stuff—some that I wanted and some that was fun to look at for the moment but I was going to be fine without. I didn't go through the things that had belonged to my mom. I'd already done enough of that after she'd died.

It was still emotional. Several times I was close to tears. At other times I felt like laughing. Once I did actually chuckle out loud. I also wondered if I'd feel my mom's presence. I know it sounds strange, but several times after she passed away I know that she visited me. There was an occasion when my computer kept turning on and off by itself. There was also another time when my cell phone kept ringing but no one was calling me. Both times I'd sensed my mom.

But not this time, and after a couple hours, I was ready to close up the house. I had a pile of things that I wanted to take with me—enough to fill a box. Nothing I found was going to change my life, but I did wonder why my mom had left so much stuff behind when we moved.

I knew the answer. She was always running away from her life;

this was more proof. I wanted to be angry with her, but I couldn't. I realized that in her haste to leave she'd given me a gift. She'd allowed me to return to our life together here in a way she never could while she was alive: with forgiveness in my heart.

Then a weird thing happened. Before shutting the door, something on a table caught my eye. It was my Puss 'n Boots pop-up book—the only book I remembered my mom reading to me when I was little. I hadn't seen it on the table earlier, but seeing it then made me smile. I put it in the box of stuff I was taking with me.

"Thanks, Mom," I said, taking one last look around before shutting the door.

Later, as my dad and I got ready for the drive back to Massachusetts, he saw me put the box of stuff in the back of the car. I described a few of the things that I'd found. Some of those items, like my Sebastian Bach poster, inspired a few stories that made us laugh. As we hit the highway, we stopped talking and listened to the radio.

There are two childhoods.
There's the one you live, and there's the one you come to understand.

Somewhere during that stretch I realized that I'd taken more from the Gray House than was in the box.

TWO

A New York Doll

My mom was one of those special women who walked into a room and made heads turn. In her case, the room she walked into was in lower Manhattan and the heads that turned belonged to Andy Warhol and his crowd of hipsters. Blond and beautiful, Cyrinda Foxe was her own best creation.

This was also her curse. Long after her best years were behind her, she still referred to herself as a sex kitten. She was so entertaining when she got in that playful sort of mood. Her eyes came to life. Even later in life, when she'd gained enough weight to make her sylphlike figure as much of a relic as the designer outfits she'd worn and then got rid of because they were from some bygone season, she still possessed that magic quality, that special *it*, and she tried to pass bits and pieces of that to me.

I can picture her striking a pose in the living room of our apartment, which was decorated with signed Warhol lithographs.

"Mia, listen to me," she said. "Sex kittens don't get fat."

"They don't?"

"No." She smiled and made her voice a soft, playful purr. "They get fluffy."

• • •

Her real name was Kathleen Hetzekian. I don't know many specifics about her childhood. When I was growing up, she didn't tell stories about her youth. Bits and pieces slipped out periodically, but those were unhappy times and she didn't revisit them in detail until her 1997 autobiography, *Dream On: Livin' on the Edge with Steven Tyler and Aerosmith*, which she wrote for the money, not because she wanted to.

It was a scurrilous tell-all; I never did more than skim it for facts. Born in 1952, in Santa Monica, she was the youngest of three children. Her brother and sister, William and Lynda, were twelve and ten years older. Both of them left home as soon as they turned eighteen. My mom said their absence devastated her. "I had no friends to take their place," she explained in her book.

Her mother was also a beautiful, Marilyn Monroe–like blond and a former model, who likely knew what my mom would discover on her own, that while beauty made its own rules, it also created its own problems and disappointments. Her fourth husband was an air force officer whose career caused them to move from Washington to Oregon and the Philippines. My mom complained of always having to say good-bye to her friends and leave her pets behind.

Six years old when her mother married into the military, my mom hated her stepfather. He was a stern, physically abusive man who hit her for any number of reasons ranging from bringing home bad grades to speaking in a tone he didn't like. "He gave the word *pig* new meaning," she wrote.

One time, when I was about twelve, I playfully snapped my leather belt together, just to hear it crack, and my mom freaked out.

"What's the big deal?" I asked.

"I don't want to go into it," she said.

Later, she told me that it was because her father had spanked her with belts and the sound brought back terrible memories.

I got the impression that her mother didn't interfere. In fact, I got the impression that her mother could be equally strict and overbearing. "I'd be in trouble if my teeth touched the fork while I was eating," my mom recalled in her book. "This was my mother's idea of etiquette. I hated eating, but I did have perfect little manners."

At fifteen, she escaped her mother and stepfather by moving in with her biological father and his family in Orange County, California. I have no idea what kind of relationship she had with her real dad. I'm going to guess they weren't close, because she lasted less than a year with him. Into boys, rock and roll, and partying, she was deemed too wild and sent back to her mother and stepfather, who'd moved to an air force base in Oklahoma.

Two years later, she changed her name to Cyrinda Foxe. The first name came from a girl who'd befriended her at the army school in the Philippines, and she chose Foxe—well, I don't know why. I'm going to say it was because she was foxy. She was, too. She had straight blond hair, a perfect figure, and a sense of style. With her new name, she moved to New York City and set out to find a new and better life.

At Max's Kansas City, the legendary Greenwich Village hangout for rockers and artists, she met Andy Warhol's transsexual superstar Candy Darling. My mom famously declared Candy "the most beautiful woman" she'd ever seen, and then laughingly added the kicker—she's "a man!" Candy reciprocated by introducing my mom to everyone at Max's. One guy got her modeling jobs, a photographer asked if she wanted to be in a movie, and the next thing she knew she was in Warhol's cult film *Bad* and then appeared in his play *Pork*.

It happened quickly for her. She had looks, an eye for fashion, and flair. She also had a deep need to be accepted and find a place where she fit in. She had an affair with David Bowie, who wore her clothes onstage. She supposedly was the inspiration for his classic song "The Jean Genie."

In 1973, she met David Johansen, the leader of the influential glam-rock band the New York Dolls. She thought David was cute and liked that he was the hot guy in the center of that fashion- and status-centric downtown world. They got married less than a year after meeting and lived in a tiny apartment. They were hard-core druggies: heroin, coke, and alcohol. She once told my dad that David would get so fucked up he couldn't make it to the bathroom and peed in his dresser drawers.

Through the Dolls, she met Joe Perry and his first wife, Elyssa. My mom dealt them heroin out of David's apartment. I don't know if she was the dealer or merely answering the door, but she was in the middle of the transactions. I've known lots of people who live that life, but it's still hard for me to picture my mom, as beautiful as she was then and as much as she enjoyed her champagne and Hermès, living like that.

But hey, look at the other New York dolls who preceded her, Gia and Edie.

THREE

Walk This Way

The Dolls and Aerosmith shared the same manager, David Krebs, so theirs was an incestuous world of business and friendships. Because Joe Perry wanted to produce an album for the Dolls, my mom got close with his wife, Elyssa. The two of them were in Krebs's office one afternoon when my dad walked in.

It was 1977, and Aerosmith had rocketed from a great band to a supergroup with the releases of the albums *Toys in the Attic* and *Rocks*, an inspired collection of hard-hitting, high-combustion, destined-to-be-classic rockers including "Sweet Emotion," "Walk This Way," and "Back in the Saddle."

My dad was the quintessential rock star, walking, talking, snorting, shooting, and living the life to the hilt. He swaggered into the management office that day wearing a custom-made velvet coat comprised of every conceivable color. It made Joseph and his Amazing Technicolor Dreamcoat look like he was in black and white. I know this to be true, because that coat hangs in my closet.

My mom thought it was wild—and my dad even wilder. She turned to Elyssa and asked, "What's that?" It wasn't clear whether she meant the coat or my dad. As soon as my dad noticed the hot blond with Joe's wife, he said, "Oh, what's that?" There was no doubt what he meant.

Steven Tallarico was born on March 26, 1948, in New York City. He and his older sister, Linda, were raised in nearby Yonkers. Unlike my mom's background, the Tallaricos were a close-knit family of Italian, German, Russian, and Native American heritage. Music was their passion. My dad's father taught piano at Cardinal Spellman High School in the Bronx. His brother, my uncle Ernie, was a piano tuner. Everyone in the Tallarico family was either a teacher or a tuner.

In addition to teaching, my dad's father led the Vic Tallarico Orchestra. My uncle Ernie played saxophone in it. At fourteen, my dad joined them on the drums. When I was younger, family gatherings turned into lively, impromptu concerts. I still remember those jam sessions as some of the best shows I've ever seen.

My dad spent summers in Sunapee, where his family owned a small lodge, the Trow-Rico Resort. There, at age twenty-one, he met Joe Perry, who worked in a restaurant. My dad loved Joe's French fries. Through them, he learned that Joe played in a local band. He suggested they put together their own band. A year later, after both had moved to Boston, my dad hooked up with Joe's group, the Jam Band, which included Tom Hamilton. Soon they added Joey Kramer and Brad Whitford, and thus was born Aerosmith.

Their 1973 debut album with Columbia Records flopped, but the records that followed went gold and platinum. Fame came quickly. So did drugs, women, money, and problems. My dad's and Joe's prodigious intake of cocaine and heroin inspired some journalist to dub them the "Toxic Twins" By the mid-1970s, my dad's drug habit cost him $2,000 a week.

"We'd gotten to a very dangerous point where we could afford all the vices we wanted," Tom Hamilton said of the band at that time. "We had our mansions, our Ferraris, the bottomless stashes. Where do you go from there?"

• • •

My mom went on the road with Elyssa Perry for the last leg of Aerosmith's 1977 tour, and there are two schools of thought about her hooking up with my dad.

One side recalled herself eyeing my dad with the calculating sophistication of a professional groupie looking for a lifetime annuity. Someone even recalled her saying she wanted to take my dad for everything he had. Others remembered my dad being obsessed about getting in her pants. "She took that Marilyn Monroe spin and had it nailed down," he said of her around that time.

Both interpretations probably contain kernels of truth, but who cares? The fact is they got together. But it wasn't like my mom gave him the key to her hotel room. In reality, she wouldn't even let him inside her hotel room. It was as if she intuitively knew all those things that were later in the book *The Rules*. Her resistance only increased his determination to get her. From what I was told, he stood outside her hotel room, scratched on the door, and howled, "Cyrinda! I love you!"

She finally let him sit on the bed, but on the condition he leave the door open. But the next time he visited, they closed the door.

In my mom's journal from those days, which I found after her death, there's a section where she wrote down the arrival time and number of the airline flight she was scheduled to take back to John F. Kennedy International Airport from the Aerosmith tour. According to her notes, David was supposed to meet her at the airport. But she never made the flight. Per other accounts, David called Elyssa and asked where Cyrinda was, and Elyssa told him the truth. "She's in Texas with Steven."

That year, she and David were divorced. In early 1978, she was pregnant with me. She filled her diary with romantic musings about how in love she was with my dad. Then there was a three-year gap between entries. "At least I have my beautiful two-year-old daughter," she wrote in 1981. "But Steven is an asshole."

FOUR

What Do You Do
with a Baby

On September 1, 1978, my parents—my dad was thirty and my mom was twenty-six—exchanged wedding vows in a simple, nondenominational ceremony in New Hampshire. They stood on a huge rock in the back hills. It was a kind of half-hippie, half-traditional wedding. My dad wore a suit, Kahlil Gibran was quoted, and my grandfather played the accordion.

My mother, who wore flowers in her hair and glowed with happiness, was six and a half months pregnant and would soon experience that special time in the life of a rock star's wife when she goes from sex kitten to fat house cat.

Before going into labor, my mom had overheard my dad telling Joe that he hoped she wasn't a screamer, so she tried to stay relatively quiet even though she didn't take any drugs. I would've punched my guy in the face if I heard him make that kind of remark as I was about to shoot out his kid. My dad probably had no idea what he was saying. Her contractions began at eleven at night, during a window-rattling thunderstorm, and my dad dutifully recorded the intervals on a tiny slip of paper that's still in my baby book. He made her a comfy nest out of blankets in the back-seat of their Jeep before driving her to Mary Hitchcock Memorial Hospital in nearby Lebanon.

On December 22, some thirteen hours after my mom's first labor pain, and with my dad scrubbed and wearing a surgical mask in the delivery room, I arrived. I weighed six pounds, fourteen and a half ounces and was twenty inches in length. From what I know, those first few months were the happiest time of their relationship. When I was three months old, my dad observed that I sang my first song, the Who's "Who Are You."

"Just like daddy," he wrote in my baby book.

Two months later, my mom reported that I was trying to crawl. She also wrote that she and my dad had played with me in the Jacuzzi.

"Mia is the best gift God has truly blessed me with," she wrote. "The love and joy I receive from her could never be duplicated or denied. Happiness has found its way to me through this very special girl. I love her as no other."

Years later, I learned that my mom had got an abortion when she was with David Bowie. She also aborted two pregnancies with my dad after giving birth to me. Why they kept me is a mystery.

But knowing that I was the only one of her four pregnancies that she kept has made me think that I was supposed to be here, that my life was destined to mean something, and knowing that has made me stronger.

"What do you do with a baby when you're a rock-and-roll guy?" my dad once asked.

Good question. He hit the road with his band and left my mom to take care of me. Her role went from hot mama to baby's mama. It wasn't very sexy. Nor did it promote the sort of secure feelings she as a new mother would've craved. She knew my dad and what he was like. I'm sure she didn't want to imagine him on the road without her, but she had no choice.

When I was four, we stayed for a while in a beach home in Fort Lauderdale that belonged to a friend of my dad while the band recorded. The place was party central. It was like a 7-Eleven; it never closed. As far as I can remember, I didn't have any bedtime or routine. The house had security cameras everywhere and I watched the closed-circuit channel on a tiny monitor as if it were a regular program.

I saw everything going on in the house. One time I watched cops and paramedics deal with a well-known rocker from another group who OD'd. Another time I saw my dad saunter across the screen stark naked. I don't remember being shocked by that, except for the fact that the crappy little monitor made his wiener look orange, and for years I thought all guys had different-colored wieners.

It was while we were there that my mom and dad's marriage began gasping for air. My mom and I moved to St. Martin, while my dad did his rock star thing. I remember my mom relaxing and taking advantage of the sun. I'm sure there was more going on between my parents, but I was too young and too busy eating coconuts to notice. No matter how chill this corner of paradise was, it was a tough spot for my mom. At thirty, her marriage was crumbling, she had a kid, she was cut off from her family, and she'd been shipped off to the Caribbean.

I might know more if I read her book thoroughly, but I don't know what to trust in it, and so I'm going by my own recollections.

I was well cared for by the two wonderful, plump, warm island women who also cleaned our house and cooked. They were the first black people I'd seen. I remember asking my mom what they were, why they were different than us. My mom explained that everyone was different, whether you were the same or another color.

"But if I'm this color," I said, showing her my arm, "what are they?"

"They're dark-skinned beauties," my mom said.

And they were. Those women were calm, reassuring, atten-tive, and affectionate. They prepared my meals, brushed my hair, fed me coconuts, watched me by the pool, and sang to me at night. It's funny; I'd been exposed to women the world thought were im-possibly sexy. But I still think of those two women as among the most beautiful people I've ever seen.

After a couple months in St. Martin, my mom and I moved to New York. She was happier upon returning to her home turf. We moved into an apartment on the Upper West Side belonging to music producer Jack Douglas. He had a son my age and I was thrilled when I discovered his toys. My mom enrolled me at the local Montessori school and then she set about reconnecting with her pals.

Her best friend was Dolls guitarist Johnny Thunders. They hung out all the time. Sometimes she took me to his apartment. Even though I was only five, I had a crush on him and flirted shamelessly. He always had a can of dried dates on the counter, and one time I offered him the can and asked, "Hey, Johnny, do you want a date?"

My mom got back in the swirl by throwing parties for all her friends from the Warhol punk and glam scene. Free to wander, I took it all in. I remember the sweet smell of burning cannabis and music playing all night. My mom typically stayed in bed until at least noon, depending on her bedtime. One day she woke up and found me on the floor playing with a vial of white pills that had been on the table.

"Where'd you get those?" she asked, grabbing them out of my hand.

"I found them," I said.

She shook her head. I'm sure she was angry at herself or some-one else for leaving them out. I thought she didn't believe me.

"I swear I found them on the floor," I cried.

"Don't you *ever* take pills or anything else you find," she repri-manded me. "Do you hear me? Do you understand?"

"Yes."

After realizing she'd been out of line, she apologized for speaking harshly to me for something that wasn't my fault. Such swings were typical. One minute she'd lash out at me, then later she'd want me to crawl into bed beside her and watch a Disney movie. I don't know that I ever complained. But one night I tried to light her bed on fire with a candle that I'd found still burning after she'd fallen asleep. She woke up and extinguished the flames before they did serious damage.

For the rest of her life, she referred to that as the time I tried to kill her. You don't have to be Freud to know that what I wanted was for her to wake up, get her ass out of bed, and pay attention to me.

I'm sure my mom would rather have gallivanted around like my dad—or with my dad, who didn't have any of her same child-rearing responsibilities. I'm not surprised she had two abortions after me. Three kids would've been way more than she could've handled. She had her hands full making sure I was fed, clothed, in school, and watched when she wanted to go out.

She had her own scene to make. She enjoyed meeting friends for lunch and hitting the hot spots or a friend's house at night. Her identity was as tied to making the scene as my dad's was to a scarf-draped microphone on a stage. My babysitter was a woman named Deb, though calling her a babysitter gives her more credit than she deserves.

In her early forties, Deb was a tough lady. She had dirty blond, hair and a raspy voice from smoking and drinking. She dealt with me through intimidation and abuse. I remember her taking me to her apartment one day and hitting me with a vacuum hose after I touched one of the miniature glass figurines she collected. I also got smacked when she walked into the bathroom and found me covered with blood after I'd tried to shave my legs. "What the hell are you doing?" she asked.

What the hell was *she* doing?

She took me to her friend's apartment, where she played cards;

God forbid watching me should interrupt her life. At her friend's, she put a chair in the hallway and said, "Sit here—and don't you give me any trouble!" Every so often she glanced out the door to make sure I was still there. I was scared shitless to move. The same thing happened another time when she left me outside on the street while she had sex with her boyfriend in our place. "Don't move until I come get you," she said.

I stood there until a lady from the building who was out walking her large, white dog spotted me leaning against a pole, crying, and brought me up to her apartment, where I played games until my mom came and picked me up. I don't know how Deb explained that one to my mom, but no questions were asked. As for me, I was too scared of Deb to rat her out.

I built up a distrust and dislike of my mom for what she let happen to me. That was never more true than when she had Deb watch me overnight. Her boyfriend spent the night, and he was a creepy dude. In the morning, the three of us watched TV in my mom's room. Then Deb got up and announced she was going to take a shower. Before going into the bathroom, she laid my clothes out on my mom's bed and told me to change out of my pajamas. When I turned around, her boyfriend was watching me. I felt uncomfortable.

"Go ahead," he intoned. "Do what she said. Change your clothes."

I don't remember anything after that. Years ago, as I went through therapy in rehab, I started to remember the incident. My breathing grew short and I was hit with a wave of anxiety that left me in tears. I didn't know why, and I couldn't get any further. I don't think I wanted to at the time. Since then, I sometimes get taken back to that place where I clench up with fear. It can be triggered by a smell, by a feeling, by anything. Then, boom, I hear his voice. Ugh, I hate it.

Thus far, I've refused to open the door to that memory. I know it's there, and I've sworn to myself that I'm going to get treatment for it one day. Then I'll reclaim that part of my life and put it behind me for good.

FIVE

There Is No Santa

I was kicked out of the Montessori school when I was six years old for pulling a switchblade-like comb on another girl after she'd hit me with a wooden block. It wasn't really a knife, but it got me labeled as a troublemaker, and the woman who ran the place told my mom to find me a new school.

I never got over the injustice of that rush to judgment. Nothing happened to the girl who hit me. No one ever asked for my side of the story either. My mom didn't stick up for me. In addition, I was pissed that I never got to pick up my ET lunchbox, which I'd left in the classroom after being sent to the office. Nor did I get my comb back. I know those are little things, but I remember them because, like so many other little things in my childhood, they went unresolved.

A short time later, my mom and I moved to Sunapee. It wasn't by choice. My mom would've stayed in the city if she could have. To her, the good life was a Park Avenue address, a closet full of designer labels, and invitations to the hottest parties. But she didn't have an option. Two factors contributed to that situation. First, Jack wanted his apartment back. Then there was the economic reality of our lives.

Without a job or any means of support, my mom was dependent on my dad, who was struggling through a low point in Aerosmith's career. He and Joe had split, and it appeared, as *Rolling Stone* opined, that the band's best days were behind them. Obviously that wasn't true. Near the end of the decade, after sobering up, my dad, Joe, and the other guys would patch up their differences and Aerosmith would crank out a string of hits that reestablished them as one of the greatest rock bands ever. But that was still years in the future. Back in the mid-1980s, with my mom and me needing a place to live, my dad couldn't afford to keep us in New York City. His New Hampshire house wasn't being used. So he sent us there.

My mom wasn't happy about moving to the sticks, where she was far away from her friends and everything else that mattered to her. As much as I immediately loved the house, the woods, and the freedom I had to play outside, it wasn't the life she'd envisioned for herself. Not living in the country. Not raising a kid there as a single mother. She didn't belong in a place like Sunapee.

She was like a Warhol hung in a barn in the middle of nowhere.

She was meant to be seen and appreciated in another way.

I don't remember how often my dad visited, but I recall him showing up fairly often after we first moved there. We spoke on the phone all the time. He called every Saturday morning and we watched *Pee Wee's Playhouse* together, talking and laughing on the phone. Each time, I asked if I could live with him. He always said no, it wasn't a good idea, and that he'd see me soon.

Soon always meant something different depending on whether he was on the road, recording, or at home outside of Boston. But his visits always filled me with excitement as I anticipated going on long walks in the summer or making snow angels if there was snow on the ground.

His presence always charged my mom up, too. Maybe she still

loved him and hoped to start something up again, but she also hit him up for money, which was always in short supply and a touchy subject. I was reminded of that constantly from the way she spoke about her car, a Saab that she referred to as "the bread-and-butter car." She dreaded the day it would break down. "I don't know what I'll do," she said.

She was so conflicted about my dad that she didn't know how to act around him when he did finally show up. Once, after she tripped going upstairs, my dad joked, "Oh, you're falling for me again," and that set her off. Another time, as she began to yell, I stepped in front of her like a referee and asked, "What now?"

"He stole my underwear and put it on his head," she complained.

I looked across the room at my dad, who was shaking his head while holding her limp panties in his hand. Then I looked back at my mom.

"That's it?" I asked. "He's playing. Don't let him bother you."

"You don't understand," she said. "He tortures me."

No, *she* didn't understand. Her fights with my dad were the result of her own anger, disappointment, depression, and frustration at everything about her life—just her simple inability to get her shit together. Since she didn't work, she slept until she felt like getting up, then spent the afternoon watching soap operas, and at night she either watched more TV or hung out with friends she made in the area, nice people who were basically her drug buddies.

On Sundays, we went to church. That was the only predictable thing about my mom. I never understood her devotion to something that she didn't appear to practice in her everyday life. Her parenting was as unpredictable. She smacked me for leaving candy wrappers under the TV. At the dinner table, she yelled at me to have better table manners; in fact, she made sure mine were perfect. On occasion she bought me toys and then took them away for no reason.

She didn't see that she was repeating the same kind of behavior she'd hated in her own parents. On the Christmas after I turned seven, I complained that Santa didn't bring me a single toy on my list, and she ripped into me.

"There is no Santa," she screamed as I cowered in front of her. "I AM FUCKING SANTA CLAUS!"

That declaration epitomized my childhood. There was no mystery, there were no secrets, there was nothing left to my imagination.

I remember marching to my room, fuming and saying to myself, "I hate her"—and that hatred, based on everything from her erratic, sometimes cruel treatment of me to the way she left me with strangers who had no business watching little kids, lasted for years. But looking back at her strengths and shortcomings and also knowing what a character she was, I recognize that she was in way over her head when it came to raising a kid in the country. It wasn't her. She didn't have the skills.

Nor did she try to learn them. Before she went to bed, my mom filled a bowl with Cheerios and left it on the counter for my breakfast. I don't remember the first time I came downstairs in the morning, walked in the kitchen, and realized that was the extent of the help I was going to get from her, but by the time I was six years old it was clear that I was on my own. After a year at the local elementary school, my mom switched me to the private Catholic school.

School rules required a uniform. I liked that. It eliminated guesswork in the morning about what to wear and made it easy when I did the laundry.

The downside of Catholic school was that it was an hour away and the public bus, known as the County Coach, wouldn't pick me up because we lived too far out of the way. So I had to get myself to the County Coach. To do that, I rode my bike about a mile into town. After hiding it behind a Dumpster in back of a convenience store, I walked down a hill, crossed a busy street, and then stood in front of the bank where the County Coach picked me up.

The County Coach was actually a large van. In addition to

the handful of kids like me going to school, it transported mentally challenged adults to jobs and the elderly to hospital appointments. All of us sat together. I had little tolerance for the
hodgepodge of humanity that I rode with each day. One day after
something happened between me and some impatient geezer, I
got off the bus intending to say "I hate these old farts." Instead it
came out as "I hate these old fucks."

"You said that?" my mom asked.

I shrugged, not sure what reaction to expect from my mom.

"That's hilarious," she said.

Getting to and from the bus sucked, but what could I do? I didn't
have a choice. The trek was worse during the cold weather. Winter in Sunapee was severe. It wasn't unusual to have snowdrifts so
high they blocked our front and back doors, forcing me to climb
out the window to leave the house in the morning.

Occasionally there were snow days, but this was snow country.
You couldn't close school for weeks at a time, or as frequently as it
snowed hard. So you learned to tough it out.

One morning stands out as the most difficult. It was the second winter after we'd moved, and there'd been a blizzard during
the night. The snow was still coming down in icy sheets when it
was time for me to leave in the morning. Unable to ride my bike
in that weather, I started to walk. It was a fight just to get out of
the driveway. The icy snow felt like tiny razor blades as it hit my
face. I made it halfway down the street before I started to cry.
Then the tears in my eyes froze. I had icicles in my eyes.

I turned around, trudged back home through the drifts, and
banged on the front door, trying to wake my mom, because the
snow was so deep I couldn't get back inside through the window.

I don't know how long I pounded on the door before my mom
finally heard the noise. She opened the upstairs window and
looked out to see who was making that kind of racket out front.
Then she saw me standing on the doorstep, frozen. From the expression on her face, it was as if all the shit she'd been dealing

with since moving crystallized in that moment of me needing help.

"Oh my God, Mia," she exclaimed, "what's happening?"

It was a good question. Bundled up, I was unable to answer. But if I had been, I would've told her that it was time for her to get off her ass, help me, and then help herself try to make the best of the situation.

SIX

Night Terrors

"Come here, Boogie," I whispered.

I listened for the sound of her running through the woods. Boogie was a German shepherd, my best friend and daily companion. She knew my secrets, dreams, complaints, and fears. I remember curling up in my bedroom with her that morning after my mom let me in from the winter storm, and I remember calling her one day the following spring and then shushing her as she hurried by my side, licked my face, and panted while I hid from my mom behind the shed that housed the generator.

"Quiet, Boogie," I said. "I don't want Mom to find me."

I grabbed her collar and pulled her close. She licked me again and nuzzled into my shoulder. She was reliable and dependable, two qualities I didn't get from my mom. I leaned on her for emotional comfort and company when there wasn't anyone else around to provide it.

We watched my mom scan the backyard as she called my name. She took a few steps away from the house and even several steps directly toward us. I held Boogie back. "No, stay here," I said, grabbing on to her collar and then telling her why I was upset at my mom. Then my mom went back inside. Boogie turned and looked at me. Somehow she knew we were safe.

Boogie and I shared the same friend, a black-and-tan shepherd named Snapper. Snapper belonged to Keith, a guy in his late twenties who rented the Gray House, which gave my mom extra income. I liked Keith. He was a typical New Hampshire dude; he rode motorcycles, drank beer, and was laid back. He was too old for me to have any adventures with, but we hung out and chatted periodically, and he was good for company.

There was another house behind the Gray House, more like a shack on stilts. Crazy Wally lived there. Whenever there was a thunderstorm, he stood outside and howled at the sky. He was like a coyote with a bad comb-over. He also collected junk. He was one of those people whose house overflowed with things, for two reasons. He never threw anything out, and he always seemed to be bringing more crap in. Things hung on every inch of wall space in his home, and from the ceiling, too; the clutter from the floor rose in stacks, like the trees in the woods.

I learned to like all types. We formed a little outpost of mutual dependency in our corner of the woods, where we watched out for each other. One day I was in Crazy Wally's place when my mom called me to come home. She knew I was in the vicinity, but when I didn't respond she turned to Snapper and said, "Where's Mia?" Snapper ran straight to Crazy Wally's house, slipped through the screen door, and nudged my leg until I was home.

Late one night the dogs started to bark. I was up watching TV in my bedroom and knew better than to go downstairs. Somehow crazy Aerosmith fans and occasionally just plain crazies knew where we lived, and they came around in search of my father. Typically, they showed up between midnight and two, about the time the drugs were kicking in.

Anytime we heard the doorbell ring at night, we knew it was an Aerosmith fan, usually wasted and asking the same question. This night was a perfect example. I heard my mom ask who it was without opening the front door, and then the person's voice carried up to my window from the front.

"Is this Steven Tyler's house?"

This time there was another person with them.

"Yeah, is the man here? We want to smoke out with him and party."

"He's not here," my mom said. "He doesn't live here."

"But isn't this his house?" they asked.

"We live here," my mom said. "Now go away or I'm getting my gun."

She had one, too—and sometimes she leaned out the window or stood on the porch and let people know she meant business. Since we didn't have a gate and we couldn't afford an alarm system, it was an effective and necessary means of getting intruders off our property. She didn't that night, but I remember her at other times firing off a few rounds for good measure.

Some people didn't bother to knock and ask if my dad was there; they just broke into the house. One night, as I watched TV, I heard the sliding door open and close. I looked at my mom, she looked at me, but neither of us moved. Later, though, we noticed things were missing.

"Assholes," my mom muttered. "Crazy assholes."

I don't know if those break-ins were because people thought they were taking something that belonged to my dad or if it was because we lived in the middle of nowhere and strange people passed through the area.

One night Keith stepped out of the Gray House and saw someone at the top of the driveway, about seventy-five yards away. He noticed the red tip of a cigarette in the darkness. Keith called for a friend who was visiting him to come outside, and they confronted the guy. They followed him back to his car and watched him drive away. The next day Keith told my mom it had been Ted Bundy, the notorious serial killer, and that freaked the shit out of us.

Years later, I researched Bundy and realized he'd already been apprehended by then. But we didn't know that at the time.

• • •

My mom also had a stalker, a guy named Settles. In his thirties, Settles was a local weirdo who skulked around town, giving off a creepy vibe. For some reason, he fixated on my mom. I'm sure it was her blond hair and stylish flair. He made it clear that he wanted to know her, and the more she refused to acknowledge him, the harder he tried to get her attention.

He broke into our house repeatedly and did strange stuff to let us know he'd been there. Once he put our keys in coffee cups, filled them with water, and put them in the freezer. Another time he used a lighter to singe little items (a lamp, the pepper grinder, the table) around the house. Still another time he constructed a pyramid of magazine photos of my mom and left it on the kitchen table.

"That fucker," my mom said when she came downstairs.

"What?" I asked.

"That creep Settles was here again. Look."

It was unnerving to think he was in our house while we'd been asleep, and yet we weren't the best at locking our doors. For most people, it's a simple task. For us, it was too much. There were too many sliding glass doors throughout the house for us to keep track of.

In any event, my mom notified the police, who went in search of Settles. When they arrested him, he had another pyramid of my mom under his hat.

But that wasn't the end of Settles. One day I came home from school and he darted out from behind a tree. He stared at me with wild eyes. My mom happened to be outside, looking right at us. Seeing it was Settles, she immediately yelled for me to come home. Settles turned like a frightened animal and stared at her. Swiveling back to me, he quickly handed me a book. "Here, take this," he grunted.

It was as if he shoved it in my hands. I had no choice but to take it. Then both of us hurried off in opposite directions.

Closer to home, I stopped and looked at the book. It was a small, very old dictionary, with a worn leather cover. I showed my mom.

"Isn't it cool?" I asked.

She inspected it. She turned it over, riffled the pages, held it upside down to see if any notes fell out.

"Hmm," she said. "It's from the 1880s. Old."

"Wow."

"Why'd he give this to you?" she wanted to know.

Good question. I still have the book and sometimes I take it out and look through the pages, searching for words that Settles might've underlined or edited out, or any other clues to whatever message he wanted to convey by giving me that particular book. Maybe he felt words had failed him. Maybe he felt we misunderstood him. Maybe it was just an old book.

I was six or seven when I suffered my first anxiety attack, something that plagued me in the worst way until I was eleven and we moved away from Sunapee. (I still have them occasionally, though they're not as bad or as frequent.) Since I tended to keep my worries inside, they were probably inevitable. They weren't traditional in the sense that a tightening in my chest and shortness of breath would suddenly seize me. Instead they came at night when I was sound asleep. Without waking up, I got out of bed and wandered into my mom's room, crying and talking incoherently.

They were like night terrors. From what I recall of them, it

> Sometimes life only gives you clues and the right answer is whatever you make it.

felt like being a prisoner inside my nightmares. My mom didn't know what to do when they had me in their grip. Sometimes it took her thirty minutes before she could wake me up. After taking me to the hospital for tests, which came back negative, she had me see a therapist, who asked questions while we played board games.

"Why do I have to go there?" I asked numerous times. "All I do is play stupid games and answer stupid questions."

"Because you have issues with your father," my mom said.

"No, that's not true," I replied. "*You* have issues with him. I'm fine."

SEVEN

Naked Nuns and the Bad Seed

When I was in second grade, an older girl named Andrea told me that the nuns at St. Mary's Catholic School could never be naked. What? I froze in my tracks on the playground, as if someone had just explained the idea of the universe as a place of infinite space, without beginning or end, ceiling or floor, and left me to ponder that picture—except that the idea of nuns unable to be naked was even more mind-blowing.

"They can't ever be naked? Not ever?" I asked.

"No," she said, shaking her head.

"How do they take a bath?"

According to Andrea, the nuns wore special bathing suits.

"They can *never* be naked," she said.

"You're positive?" I asked.

She nodded.

"It's what God said."

Although I couldn't think of any nuns that I *wanted* to see naked, I didn't believe Andrea and decided to investigate for myself. The convent was next door to St. Mary's, and one day at school I convinced two friends, Mindy and Danielle, to sneak inside with me. As I explained it, our mission was simple: to find naked nuns.

We slipped in through a side door without a problem. It was dark inside, even in the daytime. The wood floors creaked as we tiptoed down the hallway, trying to be quiet. I turned my head slightly right and then left, looking and listening for anything. Except for God, we seemed to be alone.

I didn't know where to look or what to look for. Where do you find a naked nun? The bathroom? A bedroom? Maybe Andrea was right, and they weren't ever naked, though in such darkness, how could you tell?

We continued farther inside the convent, slowly and quietly. Then, all of a sudden, I stopped and thought my life might end from a heart attack. There was a hand on my neck. Then I heard a voice.

"What are you doing here?"

The voice, like the hand on my neck, belonged to our Reverend Mother, a large, stern woman who was in charge. She let go of me for a moment; then she gripped my shoulder with her right hand and squeezed hard. Although the Ten Commandments prevented her from killing me, there was clearly nothing that prohibited her from leaving fingernail marks in my skin. I looked up at her. Even in the dark, I saw her clearly. She saw me, too.

"Mia Tal-lar-i-co." She said my name slowly, drawing out each syllable. I was sure that was so God could hear it. "What are you doing in here?"

Without waiting for an answer, she led me and the other girls to the school office, where I explained what we were trying to find out. The Reverend Mother didn't crack a smile. We got in major trouble. As punishment, we had to stay inside at recess for the rest of the year and write letters to God, explaining that we were sorry. I never did find out if nuns could be naked. I still don't know.

• • •

By the time I reached fourth grade, St. Mary's had installed a new head nun, Sister Mary Daniels. She was a young woman with a large build. I don't know if she said bad words, smoked, or rode a Harley, but she looked like the type of nun who had that in her. As likable as she was, I saw her strict side when the ballet teacher marched me into her office following an incident in class.

The ballet teacher didn't like me. From day one, she thought I had a poor attitude because I didn't want to wear pink tights. I hated pink. I wanted to wear a black leotard *and* black tights. I wanted to be *that* kind of ballerina. And because I was that kind of ballerina, I got into trouble.

It was during ballet class, and we were practicing the different positions at the bar. According to the teacher, who carried a long, thick stick and thought of herself in the tradition of a strict ballet master, I wasn't getting my feet right. She corrected me over and over again. No matter how much correction she gave me, my feet wouldn't point the way she wanted. It frustrated me, and it infuriated her. Maybe she thought I was purposely trying to do it poorly, which wasn't the case. But suddenly she slapped my ankle with her stick.

Ouch! Pain shot through my foot and leg. I stopped, in shock at what she'd done, and looked at her. *Oh, no you don't,* I thought. Then, as suddenly as she'd thwacked me, I grabbed her stick and hit her back. Mine was just a flick on her arm, nothing compared to how hard she'd hit me.

But it didn't matter. The class stopped. Everyone stared in disbelief as the teacher took hold of her stick again, turned me around, and sent me to the office, where Sister Mary asked one question—"Did you hit her?"—before suspending me.

I think I was born rebellious and independent. It was in the bloodline: my mom had run away from home to reinvent herself, and my dad was providing the sound track to those who wanted to walk their own way. Growing up in Sunapee, I felt like the girl who *should* wear all black. People in the village talked about my mom and me as if we were curiosities. We were different.

On the County Coach, kids always asked about my dad. It felt like an invasion and made me uncomfortable. Why weren't they interested in me? Little did they know that as much as I loved him, I also heard a steady stream of invective about him at home from my mom, whose favorite refrain was "I shouldn't be living like this. I deserve better."

Of course when she argued with my dad on the phone, Mom restated her case. "Steven, you know we shouldn't be struggling the way we are. Mia deserves better. She should be able to use Clinique soap." Pause while he spoke. "I don't care if it's ten fucking dollars," my mom continued, her voice getting heated. "Nothing's wrong with regular soap. But she's *your* daughter. She deserves the best."

After another pause, she let out a string of curse words. "You don't get it, do you?" she said before slamming the phone down. Then she turned toward me and said, "He drives me mad."

How was I supposed to explain that kind of conversation to kids asking what my dad was like? The real answer would've been something along the lines of "Some people love him, my mom hates him, and I'd just like to spend more time with him."

As a result, I tried to deflect the questions. When that failed, I sometimes lied and said they had it wrong, that my dad was in Bon Jovi, or else I lied even worse and said that I didn't have a dad. Eventually I learned to create an invisible barrier that gave off a very clear message: "Don't bother me."

One day in fourth grade, my friend Heather approached me on the playground and said her mother didn't want her to play with me anymore. She said she couldn't be my friend anymore. Imagine that hurt and confusion. From the tone of her voice, I could tell it was a done deal, nonnegotiable. Yet she stood next to me, wide-eyed, tense, eager, and waiting to see how I'd respond.

I was so shocked, what was there to say other than why?

"Because your dad uses drugs," she said.

"How do you know he does?" I asked.

"My mom said."

Hurt and confused, I went home and told my mom what had happened. She came up with an explanation, but I didn't find any consolation in hearing that people thought we were different. I already knew that. While I can look back and understand that the little talk she gave me was her way of justifying why *she* was miserable in Sunapee and didn't fit in, I didn't care about her. We were talking about me—and I didn't want to be different. I wanted to be a normal kid, with a normal family.

It made me resent her even more. She flipped out one day after finding a letter that I wrote to my father's sister's daughter Julia, who lived in Vermont. My cousin was my closest friend and confidante, someone I called every day and often three or four times a day. In the letter, I spelled out how much I hated my mom and how badly I wanted to live with my dad. The problem was that I forgot to mail it.

My mom ripped it up and scolded me for saying such hurtful things about her. She also explained quite honestly that she wouldn't get any money from my dad if I didn't live with her. It was the first of many times I heard that explanation, and it made me more determined to get away from her. I begged my dad to let me live with him. I told him that my mom was insane, rattling off complaints in rapid fire.

"She just wants me for the money," I said.

My dad, although sympathetic, said that I had to remain with my mom. I cried, but there was no choice.

Once a month at St. Mary's, we had to confess our sins. I loathed every minute of the ritual. I dreaded having to ask for forgiveness and then list my transgressions. My list was always long. *I hated my mother. I used the F-word. I told my mother to fuck off. I stole the neighbor's plastic frog decoration.*

Every other girl leaving the box would be told to say two Hail Marys and then sit down. I'd have to say two hundred Hail Marys.

Since we went in alphabetical order, I was usually last in line, and then I stayed up there longer than anyone else. It seemed like hours. The rest of the class waited, and waited, while I said my Hail Marys and counted rosaries. Midway through my fourth-grade year, without explanation, the teacher changed the order of confession. She had me go first.

When that happened, I nodded to myself and thought, *They've caught on. They know I'm a bad seed.*

EIGHT

The Facts of Life

One night when I was eight years old, I eyed my mom with contempt. This was different than the usual anger I harbored toward her in that it wasn't related to her dealings with my dad. It had to do with her inattention toward me. She'd left me to watch TV by myself while she partied with her friend Brian and his girlfriend, and I felt like I'd reached my tipping point. I'd spent one too many nights by myself, listening to her laughter drift through the house until it found me.

It was nothing against Brian, a local guy who attended college in Florida and hung out with my mom when he and his girlfriend came back during breaks. I liked the fun and activity they brought by boating on the lake with us and helping my mom barbecue, and normally I accepted that they stayed late and partied.

I was used to it. My whole life had been spent listening to my mom getting high with friends and being shooed back into the bedroom when I wandered out to see what was going on. But that didn't mean I liked it. In fact, I disliked my mom so much that I did the opposite of whatever she did. If she liked something, whether it was cats or ketchup, I hated it.

While she was partying downstairs with Brian and his girlfriend, I walked into her bedroom and spotted a vial of cocaine sitting on top of her dresser. It was an eight ball—about three grams. I knew what it was. I wasn't stupid. I figured she'd probably run upstairs after sharing some of her stash and forgotten to put it away. I resented that she paid more attention to the white powder in that little vial than to me.

I decided to show her. I picked up the vial of coke, walked into her bathroom, and emptied it into the toilet. Some of the powder spilled on the seat. I brushed it off with my foot. Then I put the vial back on her dresser and went to bed.

Later that night, my mom came into my room and shook me until I woke up. When I opened my eyes, I found her and Brian standing over me.

"Mia, did you touch anything in my room tonight?" she asked.

"No," I said.

"Mia, tell me the truth," my mom said.

"I didn't do anything." I insisted.

There was a limit to how far my mom could push the issue. For obvious reasons, she couldn't come right out and ask if I'd flushed her cocaine. After pressing me for an answer, she gave up and they left the room. I turned over in bed, feeling a sense of satisfaction as I went back to sleep.

You'd think I would've resented drugs. But I didn't. I grew up curious about them. They were discussed openly in my house, though I suppose there was even more said privately. My dad's struggles were public. I saw half-smoked joints in ashtrays around the house. It was there.

One summer morning my cousin Julia and I came downstairs and found glasses of unfinished beer and wine on the kitchen counter from one of my mom's parties. We finished them and shared our first buzz while we watched Saturday morning cartoons. Another time we stole a bottle of wine, guzzled half, and passed out on the kitchen floor. My mom never knew.

We were less successful at figuring out marijuana. It was Julia who came up with the idea to smoke some grass. I remember shrugging, as if to say that wasn't a big deal. We had tons of grass. After making sure my mom wasn't around, I led her outside to a distant corner of the backyard. We sat down, pulled up a handful of grass from the lawn, rolled the blades in paper, lit the end, and tried to smoke it.

"Do you feel anything?" I asked, holding the burning grass.

She shook her head. "No."

"Let's try smoking some weeds instead."

We searched the lawn until we found some dandelions. We cut them up and tried smoking them. After nothing happened again, we gave up. A while later, we figured out that we could get high by huffing whipped cream canisters. I don't remember how we learned that, but Julia and I would go with my mom to the grocery store and spend the entire time next to the refrigerator case, breathing nitrous oxide until our little-girl brains went *ding-ding-ding*.

Despite warnings on the news about nitrous, my mom laughed it off after catching me in the act at home. I remember her singsongy voice as she looked at my spinning eyes. "Oh, Mia's got into the gas again."

There wasn't anything for her to be concerned about. I don't recall getting high off whipped cream very often. It was innocent. That's how I look back on most of the years I spent in Sunapee. Julia and I spent far more time playing outdoors than we did trying to figure out how to get high. Her arrival at the start of summer came to signal that the water in the lake was warm enough for us to swim, and that meant the resumption of our favorite game.

"Should we get the purple shoe?" she asked.

I glanced into the water. Both of us were poised on the edge of the narrow dock that stood above the lake. Somewhere at the bottom, about five or six feet off the dock, was one of my mom's purple plastic high-heeled rain shoes. It was a wonderful artifact from the early '80s. A couple summers earlier, we'd taken it from my mom's closet, tossed it in the water, and spent the summer diving for it. At the end of the summer, we threw it in the water and left it there until Julia came back the next year.

"Okay, let's get it," I said, flying into the water before the words finished coming out of my mouth.

Julia was right behind me. The fun had started.

One day Julia and I were playing in the boathouse when we found a stack of *Playboy* and *Penthouse* magazines from 1981. They'd belonged to my dad. We'd never seen anything like them. We were shocked and riveted. Inside one issue, I found a pictorial of two women shaving each other. I showed Julia, with a look of disgust and confusion darkening my face.

"Why are they doing that?" I asked.

"Oh my God," she said. "What if they cut themselves down there?"

That was only our first step into the mystery of sex. Later that summer, the two of us were lying in the sunroom, eating potato chips, when Julia brought up a new subject, orgasms. She made it sound as if such knowledge separated the women from the girls. She also sounded as if she'd crossed over, leaving me behind.

"So do you know what an orgasm is?" she asked.

I munched on a chip, thinking of a response that wouldn't give away my lack of knowledge.

"Do you?" I asked.

"I asked you."

Crunch-crunch, crunch.

"No," I finally said.

She raised her eyebrows.

"Well, I know how to have one," she said. "Want me to tell you?"

"Yeah."

She rolled over on her back, pushed up her shirt, and put her hand on the area between her stomach and her bladder.

"You push here," she said. "Push right below your belly button."

"Really?" I asked.

"Try it," she said.

I got in the same position, lifted my shirt, and pushed . . . and pushed . . . and pushed until it hurt.

"I don't feel anything," I said. "Do you?"

She pressed a few more times, as if looking for buried treasure, and then stopped.

"It doesn't always work," she said.

NINE

The Problem with Cars

That fall, my mom's "bread-and-butter" Saab broke down.

"Fuck," I remember her saying. "That just screws me."

When you're an only child with a struggling parent, you tend to grow up quicker than other kids. You may not smoke or drink, but you end up a facsimile of those prematurely wise kids in the movies, e.g. Tatum O'Neal in *Paper Moon* or Quinn Cummings in *The Goodbye Girl*. I may not have been completely like them, but I had my moments when I understood more than I should've, and hearing my mom curse the loss of the Saab was one of those. I knew it wasn't a good sign.

My mom bought another car from a friend of hers for $200, a Ford station wagon. She rued every dollar it cost her. Even worse was the loss of a somewhat stylish car. The new vehicle had neither style nor status, two things she always considered in any purchase. It was the same model the Griswolds drove to Walley World in the movie *National Lampoon's Vacation*.

On the day she bought it, she was supposed to pick me up at school. Finalizing the transaction made her late. I stood on the playground with two other kids, Caitlin and her brother, whose mom was also late to pick them up. Suddenly we heard the sputter of an out-of-tune car engine coming down the street. It sounded like a garbage disposal with a spoon in it. Then a station wagon pulled up, the engine coughing as it shifted with an audible clink-chunk into idle from drive. I saw my mom behind the wheel and wanted to die.

"Oh no," I gasped.

I didn't look at the other kids.

"Mia, get in the car," my mom yelled.

I pretended that I hadn't seen or heard her. Then she honked. "Mia!"

I walked over to her and stopped about two feet away.

"I'm not getting in *that* car," I said.

"Get in the fucking car."

I opened the door and looked in.

"This is the ugliest car in the whole world," I said.

"I don't like it any more than you do," she said, nodding. "It sucks. Now get your ass in the car."

We kept the car for a week or two, long enough for some of our hatred of it to subside. But the humiliation we felt driving it through town remained strong. My mom replaced it with a Crown Victoria, another embarrassment on wheels. It barely worked and made belching sounds that were equally horrific. If it had been a human being, it would've been diagnosed with a fatal lung disorder.

We had shitty cars. You couldn't put the Griswold into park or else it would stall. Nor did all the door handles work. The Crown Victoria got us from point A to point B at least, though it ran the way some elderly people shuffle down the sidewalk, painfully slow, frightened, and always on the brink of falling.

I don't think it would've mattered to me, except for the fact that my mom dwelled on it. According to her, the problem with our cars symbolized the greater problems with her life in general. Each sputter of the engine summoned a volley of curse words and that constant refrain, "Goddamnit, Mia. I deserve better than this."

One snowy, sub-freezing winter morning she drove me to school. I don't remember why, but it was a treat. I didn't have to walk into town and catch the County Coach in the arctic-like cold. As I told her, even the humiliation of riding in the Crown Victoria was better than battling frostbite on the way to school.

As we started out, my mom asked if I wanted breakfast at Burger King. Was she kidding? Start my day with a crown, like a princess?

"Sure," I said.

To get to Burger King, we first had to pass the McDonald's. I looked longingly at the golden arches. My mom didn't allow me to eat at McDonald's. According to her, McDonald's was unhealthy. She spoke about McNuggets as if they were poison. What did that have to do with an Egg McMuffin? Where did someone who snorted cocaine get off lecturing me about healthy food and bad cholesterol?

And yet Burger King was okay. Though I was only nine, I knew there was something wrong with that logic. But I wasn't about to argue as we pulled into the drive-thru line. I wanted my breakfast and my fucking crown! I remember the wind whistling through the windows after we stopped and both of us shivering.

"Don't roll down the window," my mom said.

"Why?"

"They're too cold. They'll break if you roll them down. I'll open the door."

It didn't make sense to me. We'd pulled into the drive-thru at Burger King, but we couldn't roll down the window. How were we going to order? It was like a cruel tease. I wanted to eat breakfast. Before I could do that, though, I had to order. With the car's engine hacking in idle, I grabbed the window handle with both hands and—

"Mia, what are you doing?" my mother snapped. "Don't!"

"Oh no, I'm going to get it down and order breakfast."

"Mia!"

CRACK!

The dull sound of the glass breaking hung in the air for a moment, frozen in time. Then the crack snaked across the window in slow motion until the window looked like an Etch A Sketch, after which it shattered with a climactic pop. It was exactly as my mom had warned. Glass went everywhere.

"Goddamnit, Mia. What did I tell you?"

"Oh my God," I muttered.

"What the fuck, Mia?" my pissed-off mom said.

She said it was too cold to drive the car with a broken window, explaining that we'd freeze to death if we did. She parked the car, tightened her scarf, pulled her hat down, and got out. There was a cop eating breakfast in his car. She approached him. They spoke for a minute. Then she walked back to our car.

"Go get in the car with the cop," she told me.

What? My eyes asked the question. I was too shocked to actually speak.

"You heard me," she said.

She marched me over to his vehicle as if she'd been deputized and opened the back door, like I'd been arrested. "Get in," she said.

"Why?" I asked. "What's going on?"

"He's taking you to school."

And that was that. My mom shut the door and the cop backed out of the Burger King parking lot and headed for school. Although he looked at me several times through the rearview mirror, he only spoke to me once the whole way, to say something like "So you broke the window." Except he didn't ask it as a question; he presumed that I was guilty of the crime.

"Yeah," I said softly. "I wanted to order breakfast."

TEN

Sisters

Between the ages of nine and ten, I still looked like a child, all innocence and vulnerability, a pip wanting love, attention, and stability. But there were also signs that I was growing up quickly. Like my bedroom wall. Posters of Lita Ford, Great White, Sebastian Bach, and the band Cinderella covered the Garbage Pail Kid stickers that had been on my wall. I'd turned into a little rock rat.

My biggest thrill was visiting my dad when he was on tour. He and my mom looked for opportunities when I didn't have school and Aerosmith had dates in the Northeast. My mom never made it hard for me to spend time with my dad. She wanted me to spend time with him. But she also used those times as opportunities to send him messages or get in little digs. Before one trip, she said, "Tell your father that he looks like Freddie Mercury."

I didn't get it. My dad looked nothing like the lead singer of Queen, who had buck teeth, short hair, and a stocky build.

"Did you tell him?" she asked when I returned home.

"Yes."

"And what did he say?"

"Nothing."

"Nothing?"

"Actually, he said to tell you thanks for the compliment."

I don't remember my mom's exact reaction, but she paid close attention to events in my dad's life. She had reason to. In 1984, Joe Perry and Brad Whitford returned to Aerosmith and they went on tour. During the first part of that tour my dad passed out onstage, his drug use still a bad problem. The next year, they recorded the album *Done with Mirrors*. After finishing, my dad and Joe went into rehab. Then came their 1986 guest spot on Run-DMC's remake of "Walk This Way," a massive hit that reintroduced them to the MTV audience via the oft-played video. All of a sudden the '70s survivors were back in the spotlight.

My first real sense of excitement about the band came that year with the massive airplay of "Walk This Way." I was older, interested in music, and understanding what my dad really did. With sobriety, he was also more attentive and available. His new lease on life had a positive effect on everyone but my mom. In 1987, the year Aerosmith came roaring back with a new album featuring the hits "Dude (Looks Like a Lady)," "Rag Doll," and "Angel," my dad got engaged to clothing designer Teresa Barrick, another beautiful blond. He also finally divorced my mom.

My mom had to have seen it coming, but the reality sent her into a tailspin. It was more than being cut off legally. I think it was the unsettling reality that a decade had gone by since she'd married my dad, and while he was moving on, she hadn't been able to jump-start her life. And I'm sure she thought being holed up in Sunapee with a kid didn't offer much opportunity in the way of reinvention.

While my dad was soaring to new heights, she was struggling with broken cars, battling stalkers, and fighting with repairmen about fixing our furnace. She had neither family nor career to fall back on. She'd climbed the ladder as a groupie. With few exceptions, the future wasn't kind to sirens like her.

Even so, she didn't do anything to improve her situation. She was miserable when life only got harder for her. She groused about being in Sunapee while my dad and Teresa were in *Rolling Stone*.

> Take responsibility for your life. Don't blame anyone else for your problems. Try to make things better. The effort may not pay off, but it's more of a life than doing nothing.

She was miserable as her life got harder. That's what I resented most.

Grown up, sober, bigger, and better, Aerosmith's 1988 *Permanent Vacation* tour was a monster. Guns N' Roses opened. The excitement was felt all the way into my bedroom, where I followed the band's triumphs, as well as rock in general, with a growing zeal. Arrangements had been made for me to visit my dad at the end of August, when Aerosmith was scheduled to play three straight days at Grant Woods in Mansfield, Massachusetts. I marked the days off on my calendar.

My mom was agitated. In May, my dad had married Teresa. By August, she was pregnant with the first of their two children, Chelsea, who was born the following March, and Taj arrived three years later. After helping me pack, she sent me off with a variation of her usual messages and instructions about things she wanted me to observe, most of which were focused on Teresa.

While my dad prepared for the show, I played in the backstage area set up for the band and VIPs. With multicolored wristbands and laminates flying from around my neck, I had free run of the place, as was typical. Only this time there was another little girl hanging out with her mother. Her name was Liv. From the moment we spotted each other, we were inseparable. It was strange, as if we already had a bond.

Liv was a year older than me, and although we shared a strong resemblance, something others in the know whispered about behind our backs, I didn't notice it. All I saw was a playmate. We ran around together the whole afternoon and evening, while her mother, Bebe Buell, kept an eye on us.

Bebe was a beautiful former model, Playmate centerfold, actress, and legendary rock girlfriend who counted as her lovers Mick Jagger, Iggy Pop, David Bowie, Todd Rundgren, Jimmy Page, and my dad. Following a relationship with Todd, she'd gotten pregnant by my dad, but his drug habit caused her to flee. She then hooked back up with Todd. They split up again soon after Bebe gave birth to Liv, though Todd continued to act as a father figure to her.

But the truth was destined to come out. Liv was eight years old when she first met her real dad—our dad, who'd gone to see Todd perform. Bebe had also taken Liv, who later recalled "sitting there watching Todd play—I was so proud of him, you know, my dad being up there—and then suddenly my mom said to me, 'I want to introduce you to someone,' and I was like, 'I don't want to go.'

"So she pointed at this guy sitting by the bar, and I was like, 'Is that Mick Jagger's son?' and she laughed so hard. 'No, that's Steven Tyler,' she said. I connected with him immediately—it was almost like I fell in love with him. I thought about him all the time!"

When we connected backstage in Mansfield, more than a year had passed since that meeting and Liv was still unaware of the actual facts. But she was, I'm pretty sure, piecing the story together in her own head. Seeing me, and then noticing our resemblance, as well as mine to my dad, provided more grist.

As we ran around holding hands, a woman stopped us and asked if we were sisters. Without any hesitation, we said yes and skipped off, giggling at our private joke. That was wishful thinking on my part. If Liv knew otherwise, she didn't mention it to me. But apparently she had plenty to say to her mom. She watched the show from the side, staring at my dad. Then, at some point, everything clicked and she turned to Bebe and said, "Mom, that's my father, isn't it?"

Finally, Bebe told her the truth. Later, the three of them had a private talk that marked the beginning of a great relationship between Liv and my dad. Nothing more was said to me. Having had a terrific time, I went home without knowing anything about that backstage drama.

At home, I told my mom about the little girl I'd met backstage—my new best friend. That got her attention. She quizzed me, shaking her head knowingly with each new bit of information I provided about my new friend.

"That girl is probably your sister," she said.

"While we were playing, someone asked if we were sisters," I said.

"What'd you say?"

"Yes."

We had that conversation in the laundry room, while emptying my suitcase. In a way, we really were sifting through dirty laundry—the dirty laundry of the past. My mom explained that she'd heard my dad had had a daughter with another woman before they hooked up. But she thought the little girl's name was Amy.

"No, her name was Liv," I said.

"Are you sure it wasn't Amy?" she asked.

"I'm sure."

My mom looked away in thought. Then she turned back to me.

"Was a lady named Bebe there?" she asked.

My face expressed my surprise. My mom described her.

"Yeah, that was her," I said. "She was my friend's mom."

My mom rolled her eyes.

"All right then. That little girl *was* your sister."

"Does she know that I'm her sister?"

"I don't think so," my mom said. "You shouldn't tell anyone either."

The news filled me with a flurry of raw emotions and questions. When would I see my sister again? Could we play together? Would we talk? Why couldn't I tell anyone? Did Liv know? Was she telling other people?

My mom didn't have answers.

• • •

That tour left lasting impressions beyond Liv. Guns N' Roses blew me away, as they did everyone else. If I wasn't beforehand, I became a believer in that band, so much so that I slipped a Guns T-shirt over my Aerosmith shirt. When my dad saw that, he feigned hurt feelings. I was like, hey, give a girl a break. He understood. During Guns' explosive set, lead singer Axl Rose brought me onstage and dedicated the song "Sweet Child O' Mine" to me.

Technically, I also had my first kiss on that tour. It happened unexpectedly while I watched Aerosmith from my perch on the side of the stage. One minute I was standing in my acid-washed jeans and Chucks, still innocent when it came to spit swapping. Then, without warning, Guns N' Roses drummer Steven Adler swooped in from behind and basically stuck his tongue in my mouth, wiggled it around, smiled, and left. I had no idea what was happening until it happened. Then I was simply shocked—way too shocked to consider reciprocating. I stood there, a ringing in my head, a pounding in my heart, while suddenly feeling very different than I had a moment earlier.

I kept that from my dad, but I told Liv what had happened. Laughing, she said that Adler had asked her if they could swap pants.

"Was that before or after he kissed me?" I asked.

She shrugged, and then we laughed more, nervously and knowingly. We felt like we'd seen things we weren't supposed to. We probably had. Those tours, and particularly that one, were crazy. Though I was shielded from most of the shenanigans that went on backstage, there was no telling what I'd see.

Indeed, a year later, I was back on the road, visiting my dad over Christmas break, this time with my cousin Julia, and I was ecstatic because Skid Row was opening for Aerosmith and I was madly in love with the band's long-haired, wild-eyed, sinewy lead singer, Sebastian Bach. Julia and I stood with tongues hanging out of our mouths as we watched Sebastian's headline-making arrest on assault charges after he retaliated against a guy in the crowd who threw a beer bottle at him.

I think Julia and I were the only two people backstage who didn't pay attention to the drama. For us, it was an opportunity to ogle. As police interviewed Sebastian in the corridor outside the dressing rooms, we pranced back and forth, admiring his sweaty chest and leather pants and hoping he'd notice we'd ripped our jeans so much our butt cheeks hung out. He didn't.

Aside from the Adler kiss, my dad and Teresa made sure that I was shielded from most of the lewd or illegal activities backstage. That line was crossed once, in a *Spinal Tap* sort of way. I was in Los Angeles with my dad, who was making the band's "Going Down/ Love in an Elevator" video. After, they headlined a show also featuring Taylor Dayne (I was thrilled when she accidentally stepped on my foot) and Billy Idol. Backstage, I asked Billy for an autograph. Happy to oblige, and having too good of a time to notice that I was eleven, he wrote, "Nia [yes, he misspelled my name], if you like rocking as much as I do, give me a call sometime." Then he jotted his phone number, which I still have.

I don't know if most kids go to work with their fathers, but I seized any chance to go on the road as (a) a chance to spend time with my dad, and (b) a chance to have fun. It was different than when he visited Sunapee or when I saw him at his place. Those were lower-key situations when he hung Steven Tyler the performer in the closet and gave me a one-on-one dose of Steven Tallarico, a.k.a. Dad, the thoughtful, funny adult who made snow angels with me, told funny stories as we went on walks in the woods, took me with him when he fed the chickens, asked how school was going, and generally tried to make up for the time we didn't spend together, which, by age ten, I didn't resent because I didn't expect any other sort of arrangement.

On the road, though, he was the star attraction in a giant circus, the ringmaster, the high-wire artist, and the clown all in one, and that kept him busy. Not so busy that I didn't get my hugs, time together at a backstage meal, or some fun and games, but I knew that my dad needed his alone time before a performance and space afterward when he could calm down, do business, or talk through problems.

I usually had so much fun running around that I didn't think about him until our paths crossed after the gig, and then I got a big hug. Teresa kept an eye on me, but I don't remember many rules. I ate at the gig and slept in my hotel room. As for the other facets of rock stardom, my dad was married and sober, older and wiser. He'd written an article in which he talked about what happened backstage, or rather what had happened in days when he was wilder and his behavior was unbridled, so even as a kid I wasn't naïve, at least in that sense, though I didn't actually ever see anything go on. Nor did I want to.

But groupies were as much a part of the backstage scene that I played in as bottles of water, tables of food, and towels for the guys to wipe their sweaty torsos when they came offstage. Although Aerosmith was settled, they toured with younger bands who didn't have to say no. In fact, they wanted the easy girls.

I had total disdain for the groupies. They were ubiquitous on every tour. Like a Girl Scout troop gone bad, they lined up in Victoria's Secret dresses that looked as if they'd fall off if someone breathed on them. They waited for someone in the band to ask them to take a shower, give them a blow job, have sex with another chick, have a threesome, or all of the above.

I always wondered why they were so intent and in some cases—no, in many cases—so desperate to make that connection with someone they didn't know. What was going on in their lives? Or not going on? Some were emotionally needy and unstable birds, and others hoped for a long-term hookup, which was like buying a lottery ticket and hoping it would bring a windfall.

After one show, my cousin Julia and I were playing on the stage as the crew broke it down. As we pranced around, groupies standing out front called to us ("Excuse me," "Hey, little girl") and asked if we could help them get backstage. I got an idea. After whispering it to Julia, I picked a girl and told her that I'd help if she got down on the ground and barked like a dog. Another time, I told a girl that I'd get her a backstage pass if she mooed like a cow.

I don't know whether to describe it as amazing or sad, but these girls—and some were young women in their twenties—dropped to the floor and barked, mooed, and brayed. They were willing to humiliate themselves for a chance to get backstage. Julia and I couldn't believe it. But we were brats. We'd tell them to wait while we got passes, and then we'd run backstage and never go back out.

Once or twice I remember crossing paths with some of them after they managed to find another way backstage. They gave me the evil eye or blurted out a startled, angry, "Hey!" I smiled and ignored them. What could they do?

Even though I knew Teresa was present, I was still protective of my dad when it came to these women. I didn't like them. Nor did I want to compete with them. Trying to get my dad's attention was hard enough. Ironically, a few years later, as a sixteen- and seventeen-year-old, I used the system to my advantage. With extra tickets in my hand or backstage passes, I searched the stands for cute, single boys my age and invited them to spend the show hanging out with me.

By then, I knew all the tricks and had no trouble reconciling the double standard I applied since it benefited me.

ELEVEN

The Day the
Roof Caved In

My mom had a hard time when I came back home from the road. Questions were poised on the tip of her tongue. She didn't hide it. She greeted me by the door and interrogated me for the rest of the day, until she was satisfied she'd acquired the information she wanted, including who was out there, what I overheard them saying, and then of course how Teresa looked and what she wore.

Another time, when I was visiting my dad at his house, she made me call while I looked in Teresa's closet and read off different labels to her. I did that and other crazy stuff. Eventually I wised up and refused to act as her spy. After I caught on, I got pissed off at her for using me that way.

Now, looking back from a more sympathetic place, I see it. My mom used that information to justify her misery and complaining. It was a simple compare-and-contrast exercise. The Aerosmith juggernaut steamed across the country, Teresa in her old place next to my dad, flying on private jets and wearing designer-brand clothes, while she was in the middle of nowhere, with a car that, in addition to barely running, now had a broken window.

As those issues piled up—a broken window, a temperamental furnace, and so on—she decided we were going to move to New York. We spent a couple weekends there, staying with a friend of hers. Then one day I came home from school and discovered she'd given away my dog, Boogie. Boogie was my best friend in the world. There hadn't been any warning or discussion. I was devastated. For days, I couldn't believe the emptiness I felt both at home and in my heart. I would want to call to her, then I'd remember she wasn't there, and then I'd cry.

I remember staring at my mom with a ringing of disbelief in my head. I wasn't able to get past it. She said that she'd done it because we were moving to New York City and it was too hard to have large dogs like Boogie in the city.

"When are we moving?" I asked.

"Soon."

We wouldn't move for another year and a half. In that time, she continued to slowly but steadily disassemble our life in Sunapee. She booted Crazy Wally. Then she had a falling-out with Keith, one of numerous falling-outs she had with people, and he left the Gray House, taking Snapper, my other best friend in the world, with him. I was filled with loss and distrust. How could she do that to me?

Interestingly, in her autobiography, my mom wrote about the pain she suffered as a child from having to move frequently and leave her friends and pets behind. You'd think she would've been more sympathetic. But no, she was too mired in her own existential struggle. She wanted to get out. With or without the means, it was only a matter of time when our house began to fall apart. It started with little things going unrepaired, like a leaky faucet, a cracked window, a broken step. Then shingles came off the roof, first a couple and then a large patch. Despite the weather, that also went without fixing. Then my mom stopped cleaning the rugs.

"This is your daughter!" I heard her yell into the phone as she spoke to my dad. "She deserves to live better."

She blamed my dad, but how did that help us? At some point, we noticed a wet spot in the kitchen ceiling. It was from a broken pipe. That was also ignored. It leaked for months, and the wet spot grew. We watched it with nervous curiosity until one morning I came downstairs and found the ceiling caved in. A few days later, it fell in another part of the house.

My mom said that we couldn't afford the $800 a month it cost to heat the Big House. She had a point. With its sliding glass doors and large windows, it was easily penetrated by the cold wind coming off the lake, and I shivered through enough mornings and nights to vouch for the fact that it was hard to heat it up. She solved that and the other problems by moving us into the Gray House. As we carried stuff from one house to the other, I remember saying, "We're going to live here?"

It hadn't been cleaned since Keith moved out. Its orange shag carpet and walls were filthy. After moving in, we kept blowing fuses. After conferring with a local handyman, my mom fixed the problem by running extension cords across the yard from the Big House. Yes, it was unorthodox. But hey, it worked.

As all that happened, we began spending more weekends in New York. We stayed with a friend of my mom's, a divorcée with a daughter a few years younger than me. At twelve, I was deemed old enough to babysit while our mothers went out and partied, something I resented. Not only did I feel discarded by my mom as I sat in that apartment while she did the town, but the little girl was a temperamental brat. One night, she had a jealous fit after seeing me playing with an older girl who lived in the building and chased me around the apartment with a knife.

Later, when I complained, my mom explained that she had a behavioral disorder, as if that was supposed to make her tantrums okay. It didn't.

That alone soured me on moving to the city. Not that I was in favor of it to begin with. It was my mom who had the problem with Sunapee and wanted to move. I felt a kinship with the lake and the woods. As much as I disliked the County Coach and the boredom I felt after coming back from visiting my dad, I considered it home. I didn't want to move far from my cousin either.

Basically I was small-town. But my feelings didn't matter. My mom was set on living in New York, though to listen in on her conversations with my dad, she made it seem as if she wanted to move for my benefit. She had umpteen reasons. To me, she added a new one. She sat me down one day and explained that if we stayed in Sunapee, "Mia, you'll be knocked up by fifteen," and she didn't want that to happen.

In her defense, there wasn't much for teens in Sunapee to do other than play on the lake and have sex. But was New York safer?

Within a year and a half of moving, I'd undergo a radical transformation from an innocent New Hampshire country kid in Keds and stirrup pants to a tough-talking urban girl in baggy hip-hop clothes who smoked pot, popped pills and Ecstasy, did coke, and had sex. I wouldn't get pregnant, but who was fooling whom?

A Good Place Inside Me

I wake up trying to hang on to my dream, but everything vanishes the moment I open my eyes. All I know is it was a positive dream, and it leaves me in a good mood, energetic and hopeful. It's interesting how some mornings present the day as a clean slate. Never mind the other mornings, when I feel like I'm climbing out of a foxhole and facing enemy fire before breakfast.

Today's a clean slate. In a few hours I will drive across town to appear on an episode of The Tyra Banks Show. The former-supermodel-turned-talk-show-host wants me to talk about my past as a cutter. I was reluctant when she first asked, but I came around after deciding the risk was worth it if someone would find strength and maybe feel less alone from hearing about my struggles.

I putter around the kitchen, and the phone rings. It's a girlfriend going through a rough time with her guy, and she wants support. She's been helping him confront an unresolved childhood issue. He's a large, heavyset guy with lots of tattoos, a human billboard for testosterone and strength. He doesn't seem the least bit vulnerable. Yet she tells me that he cries in his sleep and has trouble with intimacy.

"Sexually, he's into some weird stuff," she says.

She describes the infant-like behavior that excites him, but she reserves the most intimate details. She's embarrassed for herself and feels worse for him. She explains he was sexually abused as a kid by his mother's sister.

"It's like he's a little child, trying to get his mother's attention," I say.

"I'm kind of grossed out," she says.

"Is he violent toward you?" I ask.

"No, he really only hurts himself. It's like he gets to a point, then hits a wall and everything shuts down. He doesn't know how to get past it."

"Tell him he has to get past it. Or else you're out of there. It's his choice."

"It's shitty what happened to him," she says.

"Yeah, it is," I say. "But what's he going to do about it? It can't be your mess to clean up."

Our conversation lasts two hours, and I'm worn out when I hang up. My life changed for the better when I decided to help people deal with issues involving abuse and addiction or other problems that have put them on the fringe searching for a way out of pain. I don't claim to be an expert. I share my own experiences battling similar issues, but most of the help I provide comes from simply making myself available. So many people just want someone to listen to them.

Problems take up a lot of time, but without them how would people figure things out?

As for the next block of my afternoon, it's reserved for me. I make a cup of tea, put on my iTunes, and sit on my front porch listening to music. Music is crucial to my life, my pet catchphrase being "Love, life, and metal." My favorites songs change daily, but certain records are fixed in time. A Nine Inch Nails record got me through my divorce. I found the Boston-based metal band Diecast when my mom was dying of cancer. Someone in their singer's family was battling the disease, and the band's record was filled with references to it.

I like a band called Hatebreed. According to some message boards, their singer's mom was raped; he was the product of that violent act. His music is extremely aggressive, but at the same time he tells people to control their rage and anger and channel it into positive directions. That's a good description of me: aggressive but positive.

I hardly look or feel aggressive as I lean back in my chair and enjoy the warmth of the sun. I think about what I am going to tell Tyra about cutting, and I know to do a good job, I have to put myself back in a place that was so painful I found relief by slicing into my skin with a knife. As I begin mustering the emotional energy it's going to take to go there I'm interrupted by the opening riff of Faith No More's tune "Stripsearch." Like a detour, that song immediately takes me back to third grade, back to my cousin and me ripping our jeans before seeing Sebastian Bach and Skid Row, and the other fun things we did together, as naughty as they were.

It reminds me that, despite everything that has happened and will happen in the future, there is a good place inside of me.

Yeah, I really like that song, I tell myself. Putting Tyra on hold, I get up, go inside, and turn the volume way up.

Part Two

Don't let anyone,

even your parents,

break you.

—*Davey Havok of AFI*

TWELVE

The Urban Symphony

In summer 1991, we moved to New York, leaving most of our stuff in bags and boxes in the Gray House. That was strange and disturbing but typical of my mom's disarray, a force matched only by her desire to move. In a hurry to change her circumstances and surroundings, she didn't want to bring the things that would remind her of the life she disliked so intently. I can't imagine her packing either. No, she was content to throw things in plastic bags and put them away for another time.

I figured we'd be back and forth between New York and New Hampshire, though I don't recall the details of moving day as clearly as I remember the sense of being caught up in a wave whose current pulled me along whether I liked it or not. On the way to the city, I flashed back on my mom's purple shoe, the one Julia and I dived for every summer. It was still at the bottom of the lake.

I'd meant to take it out before leaving, but I told myself that I'd go back the next summer with Julia and get it. It was a way for me to hang on to home.

With my dad footing the bill, an arrangement they'd made during one of their lengthy phone conversations preceding the move, my mom and I settled into the Regency Hotel, a midtown landmark billed as Park Avenue's most inviting address. We shared an ordinary room, with two queen-size beds. My mom's mood reminded me of the crisp, clean air after a hard rain. I can't imagine what she thought when she pictured herself brandishing a gun in Sunapee. Actually, she probably didn't picture herself like that. Why would she think about nightmares again?

For her, the Regency was a return to civilization, including doormen, elegant decor, plush furnishings, room service, and afternoon tea in the hotel's library. About to turn forty and a sex kitten again, albeit plumper, she purred with pleasure as she reconnected with old friends and familiar haunts. The people I'd heard about in her stories from when she was the Miss Thing of the downtown scene began to reappear. I met Aunt Jane (formerly Uncle Wayne County), and her other colorful, mostly gay pals from Max's Kansas City.

One morning she told me how she'd spent the previous night dancing at a show by former New York Doll Sylvain Sylvain, who later recalled her "bouncing up and down just like it was the old days again."

I noticed in her a brightness that I hadn't seen in New Hampshire. Some nights she took me with her to clubs where her friends hosted parties and DJ'ed. It conjured up memories of when we'd first lived in New York, back when I'd been in kindergarten, and she'd taken me to Studio 54. Aside from being twelve years old in a twenty-one-and-older environment, it was benign. I stayed by her side as she visited with her drag queen friends. It was fun to see her in action.

One night she took me to a bar called Don Hill's, where one of her friends performed in a band. Afterward, as we ate, a bottle of Southern Comfort was passed around the table. I saw my mom put the bottle to her lips and appear to take a long swig. In reality, she put her tongue over the top and only pretended to drink. I didn't notice. When the bottle was passed to me, I shrugged and took a drink, just like her. I got wasted off that one gulp and received a reprimand from my mom.

"You don't actually take a drink," she said.

"You did," I said.

"No, I put my tongue over the top and looked like I did."

"You never told me that," I said.

My mom shrugged.

"Now you know."

I had much to learn. Despite my mom's enthusiasm for the city, I was still overwhelmed by the skyscrapers, the traffic, the crowds, and the ceaseless cacophony of the urban symphony that was New York City. My biggest fear was getting mugged. One day I was playing with my godfather's daughter, and we went out to get a slice of pizza. It was a short walk, just a couple blocks around the corner, and it would've been uneventful had I not noticed three Latino boys walking behind us.

To me, the boys looked rough, and with a slight prod from my wild imagination I was convinced that we were about to be attacked. Soon after we moved to Manhattan, my mom had told me that if I ever got in trouble, I should run into the nearest store and ask for help. So that's what I did. With an unexpected abruptness, I yanked my friend into a little grocery store.

But steps behind us, the boys also turned into the store. My friend and I stood by the candy counter, pretending to shop, while I quietly shared my fears about the situation. I was on the verge of asking the Asian woman behind the counter for help, but the boys turned down an aisle. Quickly, I tugged at my friend and we ran out the door and sprinted down the sidewalk.

I didn't allow myself to look back until we reached the end of the block. When I did turn around, the boys weren't there. I felt like I'd saved our lives. In hindsight, I know that those boys never noticed us.

I'd barely put that incident out of my mind when my mom told me that Liv had also recently moved to the city with her mom. I didn't even ask how my mom knew that; my face brightened at the thought of my sister, and I said that I wanted to see her. Though my mom and Bebe had much in common from running in the same circles years before, they didn't stay in touch, at least as far as I knew. But my mom reached out to Bebe and arranged a playdate.

I hadn't seen Liv since we met on the road. Her visit was something that I anticipated for days. I wish I could go back and remember exactly how it felt to know I had a sister but not spend time with or even talk to her. I wonder if I ever went to sleep thinking about her or paused during the day to wonder what she was doing, if we liked the same things, and if she thought about me.

Liv came to the hotel, and I was bouncing up and down with excitement as she entered the lobby. I hurried her upstairs. Though both of us had been warned by our mothers not to say anything about the sister thing for fear the other didn't know, we picked up where we'd left off on the road, with that tight, deep, sisterly bond. It was like the plot of a Family Channel movie: two girls, one rock-star dad, two different ex-groupie moms, and a secret both girls know but can't tell the other.

By the end of that first afternoon together, we shared another secret. While jumping up and down on the beds in the hotel room, we broke one of the lamps on the bed tables. Rather than telling my mom, I hid it behind the drapes, hoping no one would find it. It was the first thing my mom noticed when she came back to the room.

"Mia, where's the lamp?" she asked, glancing around the room.

Before I could answer, she found it. She and Bebe split the bill. But there was no splitting Liv and me. We adored being together. Besides the physical resemblance, we were so alike, it was weird. The funny thing was how dutifully we kept the secret of our relationship from each other while sharing everything else about ourselves. But as we spent more time together, it was only a matter of time till we talked about that, too.

One day Bebe took us shopping in Soho. Liv and I traded smirks and giggles as her mom walked several steps behind us, instructing us to squeeze our butt cheeks, a fashion-minded drill sergeant in heels putting us through the first steps of basic training for a life in front of cameras, critics, and men.

"Girls, tighten your ass when you walk," she said.

"Why, Bebe?" I asked.

"Just because. You'll thank me later."

She was equally strict about our diets. My mom was the same way. They may have couched their anti-junk-food lectures in terms of health, but they weren't against chips and cookies as much as they were terrified of getting fat and losing the pinup curves that had landed them rock-star lovers. Next to cancer, they felt the worst thing that a woman could suffer from was being overweight.

Even though my mom had not preserved herself as meticu- lously as Bebe, they were both a certain type of woman, both of them equally focused on making themselves attractive to men and noticed by other women. They worshipped the same gods: Gucci, Saint Laurent, Versace, and Dior. And they studied the same prayer books: *Vogue*, *Harper's Bazaar*, *Interview*, and *People*.

I'm not slagging them as much as I'm remembering two char- acters and how funny it seems now when I think back on how Liv and I put up with squeezing our butt cheeks and listening to lec- tures from these rock-and-roll beauty queens about the horrors of junk food. But then as soon as we were left alone, we hopped into a store, bought chips and candy, and stuffed our faces.

That whole day, as Bebe led Liv and me around Greene, Prince, and Spring streets, darting in and out of the hip Soho boutiques, I fought the urge to blurt out our secret, that I knew we were sisters. Every time I looked at her, I wanted to say it. Several times I al- most did. But as the words reached the tip of my tongue, I stopped myself. At one point, I literally had to bite my lip.

At the end of the afternoon, we went back to her house. Ex- hausted, I lay down on her bed as we talked and played. I was still in Liv's room when my mom came for me. Liv ran down the hall and joined Bebe as they chatted with my mom. From Liv's room, I could only hear the sound of their voices, which quieted at one point so that no matter how hard I strained I couldn't make out their words.

Suddenly I heard a clap, which I now know was a joyous exclamation, and then Liv appeared like a gust of wind in the bedroom. She had a mile-wide grin on her face as she jumped on the bed right next to me and put her face close to mine. Our matching eyes and lips were inches apart.

"You know?" she said.

I nodded.

"Oh my God, we're sisters!"

We grabbed each other and hugged. We debriefed each other on when and how we knew the secret and how badly we'd wanted to tell each other. The outpouring of love was so honest and pure. Both of us felt relief, joy, and excitement. I thought back to the first time we'd met backstage and pretended we were sisters. We'd seemed to know before we knew. There was no way that could've stayed a secret much longer.

I felt like I floated back home as my mom and I walked to the Regency. If nothing else ever happened to me in New York, the move was already worthwhile. But I needn't have thought like that. So much was about to happen.

THIRTEEN

Fat Camp

At the end of August, we moved to an apartment on Eighty-second and Madison Avenue, a two-bedroom on the twelfth floor—12B. My mom painted the living room walls red, hung Warhol silkscreens of Marilyn Monroe, and then spent several weeks redoing her bedroom walls, sponge-painting them a soft pink, which was a sharp contrast to the purple and black theme of my bedroom.

Curiously, she liked to note that we were next door to the Frank E. Campbell funeral home, a brown brick fortress that was the last social stop for New York's rich and famous, a roster highlighted in her mind by John Lennon, though it would later include former first lady Jackie Onassis, singer Luther Vandross, and rapper Biggie Smalls. She was also turned on by our proximity to Bergdorf's and Calvin Klein.

In the fall, she enrolled me in the sixth grade at the prestigious Marymount Catholic School. She was impressed by both its Fifth Avenue address and its reputation as a top college-prep school. All that went above my head. I had a difficult time adjusting to my new classmates, who, as kids raised on New York's privileged

Upper East Side, were different than those I'd left behind in Sunapee. I also reacted poorly to the school's strict rules.

Though I was probably born with a gene that made me naturally rebellious, I felt like an outsider. Most of the kids had spent their entire elementary school years together. In terms of sophistication, I was way behind my more worldly classmates. I may as well have beamed down from another planet.

Then Liv left me behind, too. Shortly after school began, she went hip-hop on me. I remember meeting up with her one weekend and feeling like a dork. While I was still wearing my stretch pants, T-shirts, and Keds, she was in Gap baggy jeans, a hoodie, and was like all, "Yo, s'up," and that sort of thing.

After that eye-opener, I wised up quickly. Within a few months, I wore black baggy jeans, Timberland boots, and a hoodie, whose hood gradually made its way up onto my head and over my face so that by eighth grade I would be one of those kids who perpetually peer out from a dark corner. Soon I would also accessorize with huge, gold door-knocker earrings, red lipstick, and brown lip liner.

Years later, a friend looking through my photo albums came across a picture of me from around that time and said, "Oh my God, what happened to you?" Simple. I'd turned into a New Yorker.

Before we moved to the city, my mom had started talking about me going into the entertainment industry, and she turned up the heat on that discussion after we settled into our apartment. She had a vision that now seems to me like an extension of her own dreams and frustrations. She constantly told me how my last name would open doors, something that made me cringe whenever she said it.

"Do you mean my dad's last name?" I said. "Because *my* last name is *Tallarico*."

"You know what I mean," she said.

Yes, I did understand, and that's why I gave her such a hard time. I didn't want the kind of attention my dad had. I didn't like it. But my mom did, and she pushed me in that direction. Before I started acting classes, though, she wanted me to get in better shape. During our last year in New Hampshire, I'd gained weight on a steady diet of my mom's idea of good nutrition: Mexican food, franks and bean casserole, meatball subs, and dessert. My mom had packed on the pounds, too.

While that girth may have been acceptable in New Hampshire, where such heft had been easily covered in the winter by layers of flannel, it was different in New York. I was five-two and weighed 155 pounds. My image-conscious mom wanted to look nice for the photographers outside the nightclubs, and she wanted me to look even better. So what did she do? As soon as school ended that summer, she sent me to Camp Shane, a camp for overweight kids located in the Catskills.

Being sent to fat camp could've been a touchy subject for a girl hitting puberty, but I was happy to get away from my mom and New York City. She was also relieved to get rid of me, I'm sure. Otherwise why would she have signed me up for six weeks? But that was also fine with me.

Camp Shane was situated in the country amid hills and trees. Even though I didn't know anyone, I got a good feeling as soon as I got out of the car and breathed in the woodsy air. By the time my mom drove off, I was already sizing up the other campers. Some were seriously overweight, but most of them were like me, a little heavier than they should've been but kind of . . . well, kind of jolly.

What do I mean by that? From what I recall about settling into my cabin those first few days, the kids at Camp Shane shed whatever social insecurities they had at their schools and unfurled their personalities free of self-consciousness. Imagine the freedom of a camp where every kid is gay or Goth, from a family splintered by divorce or fucked up, or, as in the case of Camp Shane, overweight.

Without any worries about fitting in or
looking a certain way, it was liberating
for those who needed liberation, and for
those like me who didn't give a shit, it
was something to do.

The camp was regimented like school, but with sports, nutrition classes, lots of working out, and controlled diets. In fact, it was like any other diet: we ate small portions and exercised more than we did back home. I played soccer, volleyball, and basketball, made arts and crafts projects, and swam. I also had my first kiss—actually, my second kiss, if I count Steven Adler.

The kiss was sublime, but it didn't happen immediately. First I was dumped by a boy named Fred, who I didn't even know I was dating; that's how out of it I was when it came to boys. At Camp Shane, they showed movies on Sunday night. The staff put up a large screen on a flat patch of lawn and campers sat on a hill that sloped upward from the screen. It was like a natural drive-in theater, except we walked in and sat.

On the first Sunday, I shared a blanket on the hill with Fred, who moved too fast for me. Within the first hour of the movie, he tried to kiss me a half dozen times. Each time he put his face in front of mine, I laughed. It was a combination of nerves and the fact that Fred looked funny as he hung his face in front of mine, his hot breath and stuffy nose inches away, waiting for me to meet him halfway.

But nothing happened. A few days later, a girl came up to me after lunch and said, "Roses are red, violets are blue, garbage gets dumped, and so did you."

"Huh?" I said, confused.

"That's from Fred," she said.

"What?"

"Fred just dumped you." Then she blew me a raspberry.

Fine with me.

By then, I'd figured out that camp was really about boys, and I'd gotten tight with a boy that I liked. His name was Todd. He had blond hair and green eyes, which I liked, and similar to me, he wasn't that overweight. He was jolly. We didn't watch the next movie together, but we arranged to meet afterward by a large tree that was off the path leading back to the cabins. Without saying anything more than hi (we didn't even bother to ask "What'd you think of the movie?"), we made out.

I don't know how long we stood in the shadows, sucking on each other's lips, with tongue. But it was a while. When I came up for breath, it was nearly eleven—our curfew, the time when all the campers had to be in their bunks.

"That was fun," he said.

"Yeah."

"Your braces didn't even hurt."

"Good. Want to do it again?"

"Okay. I'll see you tomorrow."

Even though Todd and I crossed paths umpteen times during the day, we only made out by that tree, which we dubbed our "kissing tree." Todd was too shy and uncomfortable to kiss anyplace else. We met there every night and made out until our mouths were raw. Neither of us felt pressure to go any further.

At the conclusion of my six-week session of camp, I had to go home, thus ending my relationship with Todd. Having been signed up for the whole summer, he still had three weeks to go. On the day my mom came in a town car to pick me up, I said good-bye to him before he and the other campers went to a water park. As my mom and I headed home, I saw their bus on the highway and urged our driver to speed up until she was along-side it.

Tears spilled out of my eyes as I searched the windows for Todd. When I didn't see him, I cried even harder.

Once home, I wrote him letters. Since Camp Shane didn't permit any kind of snack foods, including gum, I smuggled treats to him through my lovesick missives. With each letter, I included a pack of Crystal Lite or I sent him a pair of socks with sticks of sugarless gum hidden inside. After a few weeks, though, I started to get over Todd. As I told myself, I wasn't ready to be tied down.

In the meantime, my mom lavished praise on me for the hard work I did at camp, which, according to her, had transformed me into more of a beauty. She was referring to the thirty-five pounds I'd dropped during my six weeks away from home. I had returned looking different, indeed slimmer. But I didn't share her sense of accomplishment. When you only eat half of a cling peach instead of a bag of Cheetos, you'll lose weight.

"You have such a cute figure," she said repeatedly.

Hearing her say that infuriated me. Though I didn't under-stand the inferences of such a comment, I intuited that I was being judged for the way I looked, something that didn't feel right to me. At thirteen years old, I didn't know who I was or what I was supposed to look like, and praising me for losing weight didn't seem right. Hadn't I looked good to her before?

In my opinion, kids like those I met at camp need proper emo-tional nourishment more than they need nutrition classes. I was a perfect example. Although I came back from camp thinner, I also returned frighteningly hypoglycemic. My first week home, I complained of weakness and fatigue. My mom thought I might have the flu or just be tired from so much activity at camp. Then I passed out twice. One time I was talking to my mom and another time I was sitting in church; suddenly I went down, and then out.

My doctor had me carry juice boxes and sip them when I felt woozy. I came up with a better idea; I self-medicated with Ben and Jerry's Peanut Butter Cup ice cream. I ate and ate and kept eating until I regained all of my weight, plus some more. My mom never said anything about the weight I put back on. I didn't care what she thought. As I entered the world, I needed to figure out who I was and what was good about me, not how my mom wanted me to look or what was wrong.

If you don't get that at home, which I didn't, you look for it elsewhere: in friends, parties, and drugs. Over time, I lost track of what I was looking for.

FOURTEEN

Learning My Part

One night at the end of summer, Julia and I were at my dad's house and staying in the basement guest room when she pulled out a joint and asked if I wanted to smoke it. I stared at the hand-rolled cigarette with surprise. Having been around pot since I was a child, I knew what it was and even remembered getting halfheartedly scolded by my mom when I was four and ate pot seeds that I found on a coffee table after one of her parties.

My eyes moved from the joint to Julia's face, asking the obvious question. She said that she'd gotten it from her older brother, a major pothead. In response to my next question, she said no, she hadn't tried it yet. But she wanted to. So did I. To me, the only big deal about pot was what it was like and when I was going to find out. A few months shy of my thirteenth birthday, it seemed time.

Nonetheless we felt inclined to hide our endeavor from my dad and Teresa, who'd already said good night to us and were upstairs with Chelsea and Taj. Julia and I went into the bathroom and turned on the shower, thinking the steam would absorb the smoke and the smell. Such a brilliant idea, though I still don't know whether it had any validity. We coughed our way through the initial puffs, holding in the smoke until our eyes bulged and we gasped for air.

Soon we were stoned. Bursting out in fits of giggles, we jumped on the bed and acted silly until we went to sleep. It was then that I decided I liked pot.

When I recalled this to my dad recently, he acted genuinely surprised. "You did that? Really?" he said. The two of us laughed at both his cluelessness, which made him like almost any other parent, and at the energy and effort Julia and I had poured into concealing something as innocent as smoking a joint, which made us pretty much like any other teenagers.

After that first time, though, I didn't smoke pot again for most of the next year. I wasn't in a rush. For me, seventh grade was a transitional, uneventful year. I was still figuring out New York, and other than my changing wardrobe, I remained relatively innocent and content to stay that way. For my thirteenth birthday, my mom brought a rum-flavored cake to my classroom.

"Do they allow this here?" I asked her, meaning the liquor at school.

She laughingly said that she thought the principal and teacher would be thrilled to have some booze in the afternoon. I stayed attached to my dad, who took me shopping or on walks in Central Park whenever he passed through town. I felt bad for the way my mom treated him. She always seemed to be fighting with him about money. Her contentiousness made me protective of him, and I let him know that I didn't blame him for not visiting more often.

I was more than ready to get away from her the following summer when she sent me to the Stagedoor Manor, a performing arts camp in the Catskills. She thought the camp looked fun and instructive. As far as I was concerned, singing and acting, indeed almost anything, was better than spending the summer with her in the city. Plus the brochure she showed me featured pictures of the camp situated in the woods, which reminded me of the part of Sunapee I missed most, the outdoors.

• • •

Little did my mom or I realize how my life was about to change as she put me in a town car and sent me off to camp in the Catskills. Several hours later, I arrived at the Stagedoor Manor, where I met kids caught up in the theatrics of being actors, including Natalie Portman and Bijou Phillips. It was a funny place. Kids showed up with overblown personalities and fragile egos. You could tell the campers who were most serious. They knew all the show tunes. Others, like Bijou and me, were there to get away from our crazy homes.

My recollections of that first (of what would turn out to be three) summer at Camp Shane are blurry. I was more remote and guarded than the majority of kids who attended Camp Shane eager for their time in the spotlight. I was careful. I preferred the shadows to center stage. While most of the kids I remember spoke about Andrew Lloyd Webber and Steven Sondheim with a familiarity that sounded as if they were family friends, I preferred rap songs by Onyx and Cypress Hill.

Despite my initial wariness, though, I made friends easily and fell into the daily routine of going to acting and singing classes. Like any other summer camp, it was more about being social than anything else. Within a week or two, I found my comfort zone among those who met after dinner behind the pool, smoked pot, drank, and played kissy-face with boys.

As for acting, I played a chorus girl in *Sweet Charity*, the production that culminated the first three weeks, and then I served as both the narrator and the professor in the second session's production of *Our Town*. For that play I had two monologues, but when it came to performing them, I flubbed both because I'd spent the last rehearsal with the camp nurse. I'd told my counselors that I didn't feel well. In reality I'd simply needed to rest from the partying I'd done the night before.

Among campers, that hangover was almost a badge of honor. I went home having enjoyed my six weeks. Whether I had any talent was questionable, but I'd learned the basics about theater and acting, gained some poise and confidence, and stepped through the door of adolescence in terms of boys and pot. It was as if I was developing my character, the part I was going to play in my life.

If all the world's a stage, who was I on it?

Well, I was thinking about it.

I left camp with kids asking me if I was going to come back the next summer. Even the nurse asked. Much to my surprise, I said, "Yes."

FIFTEEN

This Is the Life

Shortly after starting eighth grade, which was part of Marymount's high school and thus thrust me among much older kids, I met Monica St. Martin, a Puerto Rican girl whose father owned a Spanish restaurant. Along with her older sister, Brigita, they seemed to know every beautiful, olive-skinned, green-eyed Puerto Rican boy north of Ninety-fifth Street. My mom would've freaked if she'd known that I went up to Harlem with them after school, and she would've gone even crazier if she'd known it was to flirt with those darker-skinned boys.

As it was, she came home one day after school and nearly passed out after finding me in my bedroom with Victor Medina, whose father was the super in a building on Park Avenue, and two of Victor's buddies, both of them nice-looking black boys. I saw the concern on her face as she said hello, and later that night she let me know, through carefully chosen words, that she didn't approve.

"What do you see in those boys?" she asked.

"They're gorgeous." I let her digest that for a moment. "What's the problem?"

"Birds of a feather flock together."

"What does that mean?"

I understood her inference, but it angered me.

"It means—"

"Never mind," I said, walking out of the room. "I don't care."

And I didn't. I was growing up and headstrong. My mom was understanding and even encouraging when it was on her terms. For my birthday, she took me to get my makeup professionally done at the Chanel counter at Saks Fifth Avenue and then to a party at Planet Hollywood, where I screened the movie *Hook* for friends. But she balked at my taste in boys. She wanted me to hang out with guys from the Upper East Side whose name ended in *-stein* or *-berg*, not *-ez*.

That's why I hid my first real boyfriend from her. His name was Gabriel Matos, and we started going out in early 1993. We met one day in Harlem when I was hanging out with Monica and her sister, and it was one of those things where we liked each other from the start. Gabby lived on 116th and First Avenue. After school, we'd get together at Carl Schurz Park on the Upper East Side near the river. There, we either climbed over a barrier intended to keep people out and sat by the water, or, if the weather was bad, we went to his house and then made out all afternoon.

Though I was a virgin, I had a clinician's knowledge of sex. My mom had taken me for a drive when I was five years old, rolled up the windows, and talked to me about the facts of life, concluding, "There's one more thing. You wait till you're older." By the time I was making out with Gabby, I'd learned the graphic details by watching adult-themed movies on Cinemax—or *Skinemax*, as we called it—and the harder-core Spice Channel, which we got since our cable TV came through an illegal black box.

Oh my God, the first time I stumbled onto the Spice Channel, I saw Ron Jeremy doing the Queen of Anal, and I was horrified. With Gabby, I went only as far as second base. I didn't feel ready and he didn't push me, though he repeatedly let me know that he wanted to be my first. Unfortunately for Gabby, that didn't happen.

• • •

You never would've known I was still a virgin from listening to me speak to my therapist. I was constantly at odds with my mom and doing poorly in school; Mom thought I was rebelling and blamed it, as always, on issues I supposedly had with my dad. Even though I pointed out this was the same story, including the same exact line about "issues," that she'd used to send me to therapy at age six, she did it again, insisting I see a therapist again at fourteen.

The only one of my mom's points I didn't argue with was that I was cocky and rebellious when it came to adults, something that was normal for my age. I said as much to my therapist, a casually dressed woman who appeared to be in her mid-forties. She was more serious and probing than the shrinks I'd seen as a kid in New Hampshire. All of them had seemed like nice, middle-aged hippies who had me play games and asked questions like "If your mom was an animal, what kind would she be?"

"A lion."

"Why do you say she'd be a lion?"

"Because she's always yelling at me. It's like she's roaring."

Since I was more mature at fourteen, my new therapist asked more adult questions. When she asked if I had issues with my dad, I told her no, it was my mom who had issues with him, that I had a great relationship with him, that I'd begged to live with him since I was a little girl, and that I'd gone on the road with him around my previous birthday, which had been a great time for both of us.

"He had the crowd sing 'Happy Birthday' to me," I said. "He loved when I was at the show, standing in the front row. He sees so many strangers looking up at him every night. So when I'm there and he sees me, he lights up."

I had a friend named Mark who told me how he fucked with his therapist by telling him lies, and after a session or two I did the same thing. The previously boring hour-long conversations livened up when I described how I liked to go to the roof of my apartment building, twelve stories up, and stand with my feet at the edge. I also told stories about having sex with random boys, even though I was still a virgin. Those caused my therapist to lean toward me with concern.

"Do you practice safe sex?" she asked.

"Where's the fun in safety?" I replied, before going into an amusing story that I pieced together like an X-rated mash-up from scenes I remembered from the Spice Channel.

I'm sure my therapist knew that I was screwing with her. After a few more sessions, I stopped going and didn't think about her for several years.

Around that time I started going out with Eric. Eric and I met in a billiards hall, on Eighty-sixth Street and Lexington Avenue, where we played pool, smoked cigarettes, and got high on weed outside in the cavelike spaces between buildings.

Eric was an asshole, a vain, cocky Puerto Rican boy. When I think back on him, I remember he was very into his hair. He brushed it with a diligence that reminded me of the way my mom's cat constantly groomed herself. He was into himself. If I had a cold, he made me walk behind him. He made me work for his attention. Yet he was obsessed with my virginity. I suppose that too was related to his narcissism. I was going to be his conquest, a story for him to tell his buddies.

But I didn't understand that then. Nor did I care. All I wanted was to feel like his attention was focused on me. Whether we played pool, hung out in his room, or walked around the city holding hands, I wanted to feel he was into me. And I did. As the weather warmed, we spent nights hanging out in Central Park, sitting on the rocks or lying on the grass, and necking.

It was one of those nights that I let him go pretty far, though not all the way. Afterward, I had mixed feelings about where and how I'd let him touch me. I ran home and called Monica, confused.

"He wants to do the whole thing," I told her.

"All the way?" she asked.

"Yeah."

"Are you going to?"

"I don't know."

"Do you want to?"

"I don't know."

Early that spring, my mom went away on a two-week vacation to London with friends and had one of her old cohorts, my so-called uncle Lee, an aging, alcoholic queen, move into the apartment to watch me. For all practical purposes, that meant I was on my own—and that meant craziness. On the second night, my friend Lori came over and we got annihilated on booze. Acting on an impulse, I decided to cut my long hair. Running into the bathroom, I grabbed a handful of hair, called for Lori to come in, handed her a scissors, and then told her to cut it.

"You're insane," she said.

"Cut it," I said.

"How short?"

"To here—chin level."

Later that night, Lori and I called a guy she knew who invited us to his apartment to continue partying. He was a French kid whose father was involved in diplomacy with the United Nations. They lived in the UN Plaza. Lori's mother and his father worked together. He basically lived on his own, too.

It was three or four in the morning when we started running across town to his place. The alcohol was wearing off. Being outdoors helped sober me up. As I ran, I instinctively reached to move my long hair off my shoulder and out of my face, except that I didn't feel anything.

"Oh shit, it's gone," I said.

"What?" Lori asked.

"My hair. It's gone."

"Yeah, I know. You had me cut it."

Realizing there was nothing I could do, I shrugged it off and focused on getting to the wealthy French boy's apartment. Once

Lori and I got inside, the three of us smoked a joint. Buzzed, I leaned back in a plush chair and looked out the window at the nighttime sky as it began to show signs of morning light in the distance.

Later, after taking another hit, I leaned back against a pillow and thought, *Wow, no parent . . . up all night . . . getting high . . . this is the life.*

A few nights later, after wandering around the Upper East Side and the Sheep Meadow in Central Park, Eric and I ended up at my house. As we stumbled inside and I shut the front door, calling out to Uncle Lee, who wasn't there, it felt inevitable that something big was going to happen that night.

Laughing and pawing at each other, Eric and I ended up on my mom's queen-size bed, watching a cable music channel where people were able to call in and request videos. At the time, Eric was obsessed with Carmen Electra, who'd recently released an album on Prince's Paisley Park label, and as we made out, he periodically took time-outs, like a swimmer gulping air, to call the channel and request Carmen's video.

To him, her video was like porn. He talked nonstop about it, and how hot she was, working himself into a hormonal froth; and as he talked, he put the moves on me. Then all of a sudden the Carmen video came on. Oh my God, you would've thought he'd just discovered the Spice Channel. Without thinking about the significance, the rest of our clothes came off and we began to do it.

And not too well, I have to say. Eric tried to do things, and I complained he was hurting me. It was as if he decided to become a contortionist. Not that I wasn't game. But at one point, I said something along the lines of, "Hey, this sucks." In any event, that was how I lost my virginity: it was a little past midnight, and we were doing it on my mom's bed with Carmen Electra dancing in the background.

The next day I was tired, sore, and slightly dazed and confused by what had happened the night before. I lacked the maturity to process it. It had happened; it had hurt; it was over. I told my friend Monica, who told my old boyfriend Gabby, who called me later that day and let me know that he was disappointed. I wish I'd had the presence of mind to ask if it was about him or me.

However, by then I was occupied by something else. I'd always heard that you bled after doing it your first time, and though there wasn't a spot of anything on the sheets when I examined them, I still ripped them off and hid them in my closet, figuring my mom would see something that I overlooked.

Which was what happened. Upon returning home from London, she asked about my short hair. Without dwelling on all the details, I said that I'd snipped it off in a fit of boredom. Something about that made her understand. But later she found a condom wrapper under her bed. Fuming, she confronted me in the kitchen, asking if I'd had sex in her bed while she was gone, which I vehemently denied. I feigned shock that she'd even ask. Then she pulled out the condom wrapper and held it up as if she were a courtroom lawyer displaying the smoking gun.

I looked closely; it wasn't Eric's.

A grin gradually replaced my concerned look.

"Uncle Lee," I said, feeling simultaneously relieved and curious as to how I'd missed that and when Uncle Lee had partied. "Uncle Lee must've brought up some guy. God, I wonder when."

My mom shook her head as she dumped the condom wrapper in the trash.

"Jesus Christ," she said. "I have to talk to him."

As for the sheets, my mom wouldn't find them in my closet until I got home from camp that summer, and by then my virginity was no longer headline news.

SIXTEEN

Damn, Still Here

My mom was still puzzling about Uncle Lee's sloppy night-table habits when she received a call from Marymount's eighth-grade dean saying that I was on the verge of being held back because of poor grades. My mom turned on me, as if my failing grades were my fault. In return, I got angry at her, as if she were to blame. Both of us had our points, but it was a mess neither of us was capable of articulating.

It was late in the year, and I remember shutting myself in my room and bumming out as I thought about my classmates moving forward while I stayed in the same classroom for another year, surrounded by kids from the grade below me. It was a bleak picture. I looked at myself in the mirror, like, what the fuck?

"I'm pissed off at you," my mom said later.

"Sor-ree," I said, with a sarcastic huff.

"You're smarter than the grades you're getting."

I looked out the window. "What do you want me to do about it?"

She let me know that she'd spoken to my teachers and they said that I should be doing better than the Cs and Ds on my report card. I shrugged. I was unable to express how I felt, namely, why should I care how I did at school if she didn't seem to care until it got to this point? She'd gone the whole year without asking if I had homework. Why now? Just because I was failing? Wasn't it late in the game?

I didn't know what I was going to do. Feeling hopeless and overwhelmed, I spiraled into a depression. I remember being at school the next day with my hoodie literally consuming my head and face. I was trying to hide, if not disappear altogether. At some point, I decided there was only one solution, and that was to kill myself.

As for how to do it, in my naïveté, I thought that you could commit suicide by swallowing a lot of pills, any kind of pills, just as long as you took enough of them. I knew that my mom kept pills in the kitchen drawer. After school, I checked the inventory. There was a handful of vials—more than enough for the task.

Then I waited for the right time.

It was early in the evening a day or two later, and my mom left to meet friends for dinner. As she said good-bye, I thought, *Wow, that's the last time we'll be saying good-bye*.

Bristling with anger, I hoped that she'd feel guilty and responsible when she came back and found me dead. I was searching for self-worth but going about it the wrong way. Nevertheless, that's where my head was. As soon as she was gone, I went to the kitchen drawer and grabbed a bottle of Tylenol and a bottle of Advil. I emptied the contents of both into my hand. Something like forty pills. Then I swallowed them a couple at a time until they were gone.

"There," I said out loud, looking around the kitchen with satisfaction, thinking at least I got that right.

I took a deep breath and experienced a sense of relief for the first time in days, knowing that soon I'd be out of my misery, my problems solved. All my classmates would be crying for me rather than whispering about me having to repeat eighth grade. I went in my bedroom, opened my journal, and wrote a good-bye poem.

With that, as far as I was concerned, my life was done. I sat down on my bed and closed my eyes, thinking I'd go to sleep and never wake up.

"Mia!"

I heard my mom calling me. I didn't move. Didn't even open my eyes.

"Mia!"

Hmmm. I opened one eye, then the other. Then I propped myself up on one elbow and looked at the clock next to my bed.

"Mia! Where are you?"

Although my head felt as if a brick had been transplanted in my brain, I realized that four and a half hours earlier I'd tried to kill myself. Apparently I'd failed. I wasn't dead. Not only was I fucking up in school, I'd even failed at suicide. I got out of bed and found my mom in her bedroom. She said something to me, but I couldn't focus through the residual fog in my head from the pills.

Simply trying to stand was as much as I could manage. It took every bit of my strength not to crumple into a ball on the ground and cry. My mom had no idea. Which was strange. We had these dual realities going on, the story and the subplot. I gathered she was telling me something about her night out, but the words weren't registering. In the back of my head, I was thinking, *Hey, fucker, I just tried to kill myself. What do you think about that?*

I didn't get the hug that I needed emotionally, but my generally clueless mom did the next best thing given the situation. She spoke to my Marymount dean and worked out a plan in which I wouldn't be held back if I passed my finals. She also arranged for a tutor, whose help over the next few weeks, combined with my determination to do whatever was necessary, produced the desired results. I passed the tests and made it through eighth grade.

There was no preparation for the way I felt when I returned to Sunapee the next year. It was December 1993, and my dad wanted to celebrate my fifteenth birthday and have a family Christmas. He invited Liv and me to spend vacation with him and Teresa, Chelsea, and Taj. It was my first time going back home since my mom and I had left, and I was excited. But nothing could've lived up to my expectations.

The house was now used for vacations and holidays. Teresa had redecorated, something that was sorely needed, but it was still jarring to find the rooms looking so different. The strangest thing was the unfamiliarity of the familiar. All my references had been changed enough to throw me off. I felt like someone was playing a joke on me. I wanted to ask what had happened to my house.

On my birthday, my dad took Liv and me out for a drive. When we got back, I walked inside the house and Teresa, my sister and brother, and several old friends of mine that my dad had rounded up yelled surprise. I enjoyed the attention and appreciated the effort, but it didn't feel right. I understand now. I was struggling with the emotional confusion of being back, wishing I had a home and a family.

Then there was Liv, who I loved and wanted to connect with the way we always had in the past. But now, at sixteen, she'd changed, too. I should've expected as much, and I would've been more accepting if someone had explained that she hadn't changed as much as she'd grown up. She also didn't carry around my same anger. She'd recently gone through paternity tests, and then suddenly she was legally in the family and also in my dad's videos, everything I'd wanted—or thought I'd wanted.

She dressed differently, too. While I was still in hip-hop black, she had taken to designer clothes that were casual but hip. She looked gorgeous. She is gorgeous. But in my state of mind, everything bugged me. I thought Liv over-tweezed her eyebrows and talked about makeup as if it were as essential as air. It was all stuff I was hypersensitive to because of my mom.

Then one afternoon my dad wanted to take a family picture. Liv made everyone wait while she applied some under-eye foundation. It was normal sixteen-year-old girl behavior. I was appalled. It put me in a mood, and I remember thinking, *Ugh, I'm so not into this. I don't even want to be here.*

Despite those feelings, the opposite was true. I didn't want to be anywhere but there. It was home. On the day I had to go back to the city, I went to say good-bye to my little sister, Chelsea, but I couldn't find her. I searched inside and out. As I walked beyond the house, I flashed back to the way my mom used to search for me. I almost felt as if I was looking for myself.

Ironically, I found Chelsea sitting in the same spot where I'd played at her age. She asked if I could stay. She had no idea how much I wanted to.

Fast-forward five months. It was toward the end of ninth grade, and I got in trouble at school for fighting with another girl. Except that I hadn't been fighting. I'd been in the back of the classroom with three girls, and we were pushing each other and laughing. But one of the girls' mother, who was at school for some reason, looked inside the classroom, thought her daughter was crying, and all hell broke loose.

Singled out as the instigator, I was sent to the Upper School principal's office. After questioning me, she called in the head nun to mete out the discipline. I had to tell the story all over again. She didn't believe me. She thought I was a troublemaker. A stoner, yes, I would've copped to that. But a troublemaker, no, that wasn't me. Yet the nun's questions showed that not only did she think I was guilty of fighting as charged, she also intimated that the real issue was that I hung out with the black and Puerto Rican scholarship girls.

Despite the pressure Mother Whatshername put on me—and believe me, when you have a stern-faced nun glaring at you, you feel pressure—I refused to admit being guilty of anything. If I'd been in a fight, I would've admitted it. But it wasn't true. So as she came down harder on me, and with the principal looking on, I eventually lost my patience and told the nun to fuck off.

Mistake. I knew it was wrong to say that to a nun. But I didn't care. She was acting very un-nun-like.

After the words came out of my mouth, the nun froze. Incredulous. Angry.

"What did you say?" she asked.

I had nothing left to lose.

"I said you can go fuck yourself."

I was suspended from attending senior graduation, the big year-end event that all grade levels looked forward to attending. My mom flipped out and made me take in a letter of apology to the nun. Although I delivered the note, it said that my mom had forced me to write the apology, that I didn't believe a word I'd written, and that, if she really cared to know my opinion, well, I thought the school's religious teachings were a crock. In conclusion, I ranted that masturbation wasn't a sin, that she ought to try it, and that most of all, she ought to try practicing forgiveness—something the school also preached!

I never heard her response directly, but I wasn't surprised when my mom came into my bedroom steaming mad and said that the school had called and said that I wasn't allowed to return.

"What the fuck, Mia?"

That was exactly what I thought. What the fuck?

SEVENTEEN

What Drugs
Do You Have?

At the end of June, as New Yorkers prepared for their summer exodus from the city, I went to acting camp at Stagedoor Manor. Although I told my mom that this third summer session was going to be my last, I knew going there was the perfect antidote to the mess at Marymount. Nine weeks at camp (yes, I'd tacked on three more weeks since my first year) would erase all of my unpleasant memories of school.

It would probably kill a few million brain cells, too, but that was the point of camp, wasn't it? It was for me.

As a veteran camper, I arrived fully prepared. I brought three trunks: one full of clothes, one full of food, and one full of drugs and alcohol.

As always, I was one of the first campers to arrive. I always left home early and got to camp early. My dorm room had three girls in it. I took the single and left the bunk bed for the other two girls. Before I unpacked, Bijou Phillips bounded into the cabin. She jumped on top of one of my trunks, which I'd just lifted onto my bed, and perched there like a tigress.

"What drugs do you have?" she asked.

I remember looking at Bijou, who was a year or two younger than me, and thinking, *Poor child*. Compared to her, I saw myself as an old soul—and felt like one. I was also living like one.

I pushed Bijou off the trunk and showed her what was inside. I'd brought a bag of quaaludes, a bag of E, and four large Poland Spring water bottles filled with vodka. I'd also brought a little canteen, which, over the ensuing weeks, I would fill at lunchtime with cranberry juice and vodka and walk around the rest of the day blitzed. Basically, I lived that summer on Cup Noodles and vodka.

Which explains why I can't recall the plays that were staged that summer, though I remember being cast in something that required me to come onstage covered with twigs and leaves. I wore a bikini and prepared by rolling around in dirt. But I wasn't at camp to act; I was there to party. I used to sneak cigarettes in a little room underneath the main theater. One day I was caught and sent to the main office, where a head counselor lectured me about rules.

She struck me as stern but not too upset. Then, after her talk, she told me to follow her out back, where she offered me a cigarette. Hey, it was a camp of frustrated and wannabe actors; everyone was a little bit naughty. On the night before the parents' visiting day, there was a girl who, like me, was the daughter of a famous rock singer, and she got so drunk that she passed out. As she slept, a bunch of us drew crude and funny pictures all over her with markers.

I wish I knew what happened to her on parents' day, but we kept our distance. What we drew on her was *that* embarrassing. My own father came out that day. For me, there was nothing better—or worse. It was actually a mixed blessing; while I savored the time I was able to spend with him, I blanched at the ruckus his presence caused among the other campers. All their preening and vying for his attention encroached on the time that I got to spend with him.

It was during one such moment when I was frustrated by the

interruptions that I turned toward my dad, who was wearing one of his colorful getups, and gave him one of those up and down looks, from head to toe, that let him know I was fed up.

"What about just wearing a suit sometime?" I asked.

My dad gave me one of his looks and said, "Come on." He was right; I knew better than that.

On the night of the staff talent show, always one of the high points at camp, I hooked up with Josh, a boy who'd done acid for eight straight months before camp. By summer, his brain was curdled. But he was cute. Midway through the show, I took him into the main theater's downstairs room, the same room where I snuck cigarettes, and we fooled around. It was trippy doing it while hearing the counselors singing and dancing only a few feet above us.

Our relationship was short-lived, maybe a week or two. For the rest of camp, I made out with a bunch of boys and fooled around with a few of them. My last year at camp, I was determined to have fun, make memories, and leave a reputation. I did that to the hilt. It was a role I played well. But that part didn't serve me well over the long haul. When I think back on those days, I see that the drugs were numbing and the sex was easy and empty. I left unsatisfied.

What I craved were meaningful connections, the kind of friendships and relationships that would make me feel whole and confident, and those, as I'd realize many years later, were much harder to make.

After camp, I returned home feeling as if I'd been through something. It was only the start. My mom enrolled me in the Professional Children's School, a coed school for working kids whose two hundred students included actors, musicians, dancers, ice-skaters, and thirteen-year-old national chess master Josh Waitzkin, who was the subject of Steven Zaillian's movie about his life, *Searching for Bobby Fischer*.

Why that school? After three summers of acting camp and two years of intermittent classes, my mom thought I should go to a school that was more about acting. She probably also saw herself in competition with Bebe and Liv, who'd landed a part in a movie after generating some buzz following her appearance with Alicia Silverstone in Aerosmith's video for "Crazy."

As for me, I was typically nonplussed. I can't say that I wanted to go, but I didn't not want to do it either. I simply didn't argue.

Then I found out it was a convenient fit. Kids were either preternaturally grown-up, ambitious, working and living in their own world of landing jobs and launching careers, or they were screwups. In both cases, academics were secondary to agents, managers, and movies in production. Many also smoked, drank, were sexually active, and kept up on all the Hollywood gossip. It reminded me of camp.

You could sign out whenever you wanted by saying you had an audition. Notes from parents or agents weren't required. Several times a week I left school for "auditions," which was code for meeting up with friends at the Sheep Meadow in Central Park and getting high. It was around this time that I tried acid. I was with my friend Lori and her boyfriend Andy. One night we met his sister and a friend of hers for dinner at a coffee shop, and he gave me two tabs of acid, which were tiny specs of paper smaller than my fingernail.

"There's a drop on each paper," he said.

I'd already done Ecstasy, pot, pills, and booze. Acid seemed like the next logical amusement. We were all going to do it together, but we split up after dinner. But a short time later, Andy called and told me to meet them at a party downtown.

"Did you do the acid?" he asked.

"Half of one," I said. "But I'm not feeling anything. What's supposed to happen? I don't know what it does."

"It gets you fucking high," he said, laughing. "Get your ass down here."

Impatient to feel the effects, I swallowed the other half of the tab and looked for a taxi. A few minutes later, as I sat in the back of a yellow cab heading to the Lower East Side from my Upper East Side neighborhood, I started to feel the powerful effects of the acid. It was like a tingling in my head, and then I spaced. I caught myself staring intensely at the thick glass divider, as if I could see its different layers. I wondered how hard I needed to punch to shatter it.

A moment later, I wondered what it would be like if I stabbed the driver and hacked up his body. Then, just as suddenly, I snapped out of that murderous reverie and realized I was sky-high.

"Oh my God, this is insane," I said out loud. "I'm tripping."

"Excuse me?" the driver asked.

"Nothing," I said, trying to keep it together while looking out the window at a cityscape full of cotton candy towers and swirling lights.

I was saying "whoa" to no one in particular as I got out of the cab. I went into the apartment building and found Lori, Andy, and his sister in the midst of this roaring party. The place was full of people tripping on one thing or another. With music filling every room, it was like a rave in someone's apartment. All of us took our second hits of acid. Pretty soon I was fixated on a guy.

"Look at him!" I said to Lori and Andy and his sister.

"What?" Andy asked.

"That guy?" his sister chimed in, fully aware of what had transfixed me—a guy with a thick, black unibrow.

"Yeah," I said. "Look at his eyebrow."

"Oh my God," Rachel said, covering her face with her hands. "It's one, not two—and it goes across his forehead."

"It's a full-on fucking caterpillar," I said, laughing. "I'm so high, I'm scared of it."

"We better hide before it eats us," Andy said.

That struck all of us as hysterically funny. We crumpled to the floor in laughter. Then we crawled under the dining room table, where we sat, feeling safe. Just in time, too. A fight broke out between some jocks and some punks and ravers. We watched for a few minutes, then snuck outside, where we climbed a tree and gazed from that vantage as the fight from the party spilled onto the sidewalk.

Eventually I climbed down and went home, though I don't think I really came down for years.

EIGHTEEN

Sweet 16

For my sixteenth birthday, my mom pulled out all the stops. She bought a new designer outfit, got her hair done by Oscar Blandi, and booked us rooms for the night at the Ritz-Carlton. My dad was picking up the tab, and she delighted in spending his money. She planned a party at the Rouge Club, where the guest list included Joey Ramone and singer Tom Jones. Photos were taken by legendary paparazzo Ron Galella. One of my friends turned to me at one point and asked, "Who are these people?" I laughed and pointed at my mom. "She invited them."

I didn't mind. The party was about having fun, and it was fun. My dad was there. So was Liv, who looked radiant. And Chelsea, who you could see was on her way to becoming the latest Tyler beauty. Surrounded by family, I blew out the candles on a three-tiered white cake decorated with purple dolphins that was delicious. My dad mugged for the camera as I fed him a piece. The photographer also snapped me with my parents together, one on each side of me, kissing my cheeks.

Later, my mom went through those photos as if she were editing a magazine layout. My impression at the time was that the party had been mostly about her putting it together and then getting it mentioned in the papers and magazines so she could see her name in bold again. It took me years before I could overlook her neediness in that department and fully appreciate what it meant to have the whole family together. I made it through the night without getting high. Sober, I beamed as I opened a gift from my friends, a thick chain with a small padlock. It was so punk and dirty. I loved wearing it with Gucci dresses.

At home the day after the party, I got a special delivery—sixteen dozen red roses. The delivery guy made two trips from his van. The card read, "Happy Birthday, Love Axl Rose." For nearly two weeks, my bedroom smelled like a flower shop. All I wanted to do was lie on my bed and inhale the perfumed air.

But my life would not stay a bed of roses. The gathering of family and feeling of connectedness that made my birthday so special faded about the same time I had to throw out the flowers. Then it was back to reality, the daily challenge to find meaning, substance, and structure where none seemed to exist. Through school, I became friendly with a famous child actor and his family.

Altogether, there were seven kids, and they resided in three neighboring apartments in a building next to the school. The teenagers had the same level of parental supervision as me, which was basically none. Their place was a safe haven for meeting after school and playing video games, drinking forties, and getting high. I was closest with the oldest, an eighteen-year-old who'd already graduated.

One day he gave me a box of tiny liquor-filled chocolate bottles. There were forty-eight of the little bottles in the box. I took them to school, sat in the back of the classroom, and methodically bit off the tops, guzzled the liquor, and spit out the chocolate. I was buzzed before noon. Since this guy was out of school, I skipped out of classes to spend the afternoon with him. We watched movies, smoked pot, ordered in food, and had sex. When we got bored, we dropped acid and ran around town.

We were like the aimless, unsupervised, booze-drinking, drug-taking, sex-having, sad-eyed, disenfranchised teens that fascinated filmmaker Larry Clark in his movie *Kids*. One of my friends actually was in it. I was blindsided a couple months later when the oldest brother called from a vacation in Montana and said that he was going back to his old girlfriend. Crushed, I hung up and cried. I'd lost one of my best friends.

The breakup exposed the part of me that my tough-girl exterior tried to protect, my fragile heart. Without the grounding of a strong and centered family, I depended on friends to anchor me, and this news sent me adrift. Five years later, I was at a Chemical Brothers concert and ran into him, and he gave me a warm embrace. I was surprised at how vulnerable I felt at seeing him again.

"You broke my heart," I said.

After hearing my story, he shook his head.

"I had no idea I did all that," he said.

Midway through tenth grade, my friend Andy and several of his buddies came over one night and introduced me to coke. By then, I'd done my share of pot, Ecstasy, and acid, but somehow cocaine had eluded me until then. Then Andy dumped out a tiny mound of white powder on a small mirror, deftly cut it into thin lines, and handed me a small metal straw.

"Get ready to blast off," he said, before instructing me how to snort the lines up my nose.

After that first time, I had found my new favorite drug. In addition to the thrill of the initial rush, coke filled me with a warmth and self-confidence that I ordinarily lacked. It made me feel on top of the world. My embrace of coke also coincided with my introduction to Michelle, a girl at school who became my new best friend. Elle, as I called her, was a short Italian blonde. Her scratchy voice and sassy personality reminded me of Taylor Dayne.

We were coke buddies. Doing coke made me warm, loving, and talkative. It sent Elle rocketing in the opposite direction. She turned inward and became paranoid and obsessive. I can still picture us locked in my bedroom. While I blabbered on and on, she cleaned the table and checked the door after every line.

I kept my coke on a shelf in my bedroom in a Where's Waldo coin bank. It was a little box filled with Waldo-related things, and you had to find Waldo inside. There was a secret spot where I kept my straws and vials. I also bought a Barbie kitchen set for the tiny spoons, cups, and saucers. They were perfect for coke. There was something twisted about two teenage girls using children's toys to do coke.

My mom had a friend named Rick, who also wanted to be my friend. In his mid-twenties, he partied with my mom and also figured out that I was hoovering my share of South America. He gave me a key to his apartment on Seventy-fifth and Madison so that my friends and I could use it as a safe place to do coke. His interest? If he was there, he got free coke and the chance to eye-fuck pretty teenage girls.

We weren't any better. If we were out of coke, Elle or I or someone else in our crowd would suggest going to Rick's to check out his stash. We knew he wouldn't turn down the chance to have pretty sixteen-year-old girls bending over his coffee table as they did lines. Yes, it was creepy, but there were benefits all around.

One morning before classes, Elle told me that her best friend since second grade was spending the day at the school. I'd thought I was her best friend. Hearing her use that phrase to describe someone else irritated me. When I saw her with Gillian Goldstein, I got jealous and ignored both of them through the morning.

At lunch, one of the school's administrators asked if I'd show a potential new student around the school. I said yes. That girl turned out to be Gillian.

Reluctantly, I agreed to give her a tour. As I guided her through the day, we chatted, and by my last two classes I thought she was cool and understood why Elle liked her so much. After school, she tagged along when Elle and I went to a nearby park to get high and hang out. The park was actually a landscaped square within a development of buildings on Sixtieth and Columbus, hidden from the street, and our safe haven. Not even the security guard turned his head when we lit up.

The funny thing was, no one had any pot. After a brief discussion, Gillian and I were assigned to get a couple dime bags. We got in a cab and went up to the Jamaican record store at 103rd and Amsterdam. On the drive uptown, I noticed Gillian had cans of paint in her bag. I found out she was a graffiti artist. I noticed her clothes: baggy jeans, a tattered jacket, and a cap. She looked a lot cooler than she had at school.

And she was. At the record store, she picked up on my hesitancy in dealing with the guy behind the counter. I didn't tell her, but I hated buying drugs and tried whenever possible to avoid it. I knew if anything ever happened, it would make news because of my dad. I didn't want to embarrass my dad like that. So I was relieved when Gillian stepped forward and negotiated the deal. When the guy gave her the pot, she dropped it in her bag with total nonchalance.

"Is dat it?" the guy asked.

"Yeah, thanks," she said.

"Cool."

She grabbed her bag, took my arm, and before turning toward the door threw the guy a look and said, "Good looking out."

Wow. *Good looking out.* That phrase grabbed my attention. She said it without any inflection or pause. Just those three words. Letting them hang in the air, like a ring of smoke. *Good looking out.* I stared admiringly at her as she flagged down a cab and we got in for the drive downtown. Although I'd only met her that day, I knew we were going to be good friends. She was one cool chick.

On the way back to the park, we stopped at the neighborhood deli and bought some chips and Doritos, then spent the rest of the afternoon smoking the pot and munching out. I told Elle that I was crazy about Gillian, or Goldstein, as I'd already started calling her.

It turned out Goldstein wasn't into partying the way Elle and I were. She declined anything stronger than a joint. That slowed down our friendship since Elle and I were occupied by our coke habit.

The drug had a transformative effect on Elle and myself. Our clothes provided the most obvious evidence. Not long after we started doing it, we traded our baggy hip-hop clothing for designer labels like Gucci, Pucci, and Betsey Johnson, where I received a discount for having gone with my dad to one of their events. On most mornings, we hit the makeup counter at Bloomingdale's or Henri Bendel, and we reapplied at night before they closed.

Decked out and made up, we hit the clubs at night. Suddenly we weren't watching TV; we were starring in our own exciting, superficial dramas behind the velvet ropes. Although underage, we had no problem getting past the doormen at the hottest clubs in the downtown scene. We weren't the only under-twenty-one-year-olds there either. The gossip columns in the papers were routinely full of stories about fifteen-year-old Bijou's antics, like the time she was at Spy and supposedly snipped a guy's finger with a cigar cutter. In truth, it was just a nick.

But that sort of stuff went on every night of the week. We got to be friends with the club owners and the doormen, and it didn't matter how old we were. They let us in. We got the clubs press. In the meantime, we were blasted. Elle and I carried around little juice boxes filled with coke, pretending to drink out of them when in reality we'd take hits through the straw. Someone had showed us how to heat up the top until the glue melted, open up the box, then fill it with coke and seal it back up. No one ever suspected what was really inside. But that's how we stayed up all night.

Elle laughed when I showed her what my dad had given me for Christmas. It was a ring with a large mirror on it.

"He doesn't know, does he?" she said, shaking her head.

"Obviously not," I replied.

We laughed at how clueless our parents were.

"It's another thing for your Where's Waldo box," she said.

She was right, too. By then, my paraphernalia collection also included a Hello Kitty shooter. With a twist of the head, out popped a single hit of coke. When I think back on that, there was something so wrong about the way even the objects of our childhood had been corrupted by the drug culture. Likewise the way I spelled out my name in coke on a large glass plaque my dad had received years earlier for the song "Dream On." I was being belligerent.

Around this time, Elle and I also got into rollerblading. Our need for speed wasn't confined to coke or clubs. We used to race up and down Manhattan, from Harlem to Wall Street, carrying small plastic baggies with straws in them. Every so often we made pit stops at restaurants, stores, cabs, or pay phones, took a couple hits from our stash, and then raced back into the river of humanity populating the sidewalks. Sometimes we actually had destinations. Most of the time we just wanted to see how fast and far we could go.

NINETEEN
A Scary Sight

Where was my mom? In contrast to my globe-trotting, concerned but long-distance father, she was rooted at home, a woman who gave the impression of being always busy with projects and social events, plugged in and hip, and yet she was a totally disengaged parent. She RSVP'd to art gallery openings and dashed out many an evening to see some "downtown NYC punk band," as she described them to me. Typically, I caught up with her as we crossed paths in the early evening as she did her makeup and I came in for a breather between school and clubs.

She rarely asked about school unless I was in trouble. She didn't help with homework, quiz me before tests, or ask what I had learned. In retrospect, that was a good thing; if she had probed, I would've been easily busted. As generous as my dad was to me with his credit card, she complained of not having any money. She was always in and out of court with him about child support and alimony, and if she wasn't in court, she was threatening to take him to court.

I hated her for that. She was capable of working, of doing so much more, but she never tried to reinvent herself. Ultimately it would prove such a waste, because she had talent, vision, a sense of humor, and just so much more to offer than she let herself. She occupied herself with projects around the house. She painted the walls, moved furniture, did little projects, or returned clothes and bought new stuff. Looking back, she did a masterful job of avoiding the real issues of her life. She didn't cook, unless you call heating up takeout from EAT cooking.

She didn't question me when I was high either. She didn't know I was high and since I didn't have a curfew, she didn't have reason to ask. What an earful she would've gotten if she had. One night I came home and she asked what I'd been up to. "Nothing," I said, though earlier in the day I'd been involved in a pushing-and-name-calling fight at school with a couple girls after they'd called Elle a "clown" for wearing too much makeup.

I was still laughing when I got home.

"What's so funny?" my mom asked.

"Nothing," I said, even though I was thinking about how, following the fight at school, I'd turned to Elle and said, "You know, you do look like a clown."

Another night Elle raced into our apartment, barely saying hi to my mom on her way to my room. She shut the door and stared at me, breathless with excitement.

"What?" I asked.

She put two vials on my table. Each was an eight ball—a total of seven grams of cocaine. She told me our dealer had given them to her for free.

"Free?" I said.

"He just wanted me to show him my tits," she said.

I didn't know for sure, but I sensed more was involved than Elle lifting her shirt. The next time I got blow from that dealer, he started talking to me with his face way too close to mine. The feel of his breath on my cheeks made me want to duck and/or gag. Then he put his hand on my leg and asked me out. I told him no, grabbed my stuff, and got the hell out of his car. I knew better.

• • •

On the verge of taking a dangerous turn, Elle was also an actress. She knew that I was semi-serious about trying to get work, if only because school surrounded me with kids who had careers. My effort was more semi than serious, though. I took lessons from a woman with her own acting studio in midtown. In reality, they were more gab sessions than lessons. After warming up with acting exercises, she would find a reason to break for a cigarette, and then as both of us smoked, she would ask me to tell her about the latest exploits of my wayward youth.

One day Elle took me to see her agent and they signed me. That was thrilling, to be wanted and described as having potential. No one had given me that kind of positive feedback. My mom thought it was a step in the same direction as Liv, an open door to a career. I have to admit that I enjoyed her taking an interest in my life. That was new. But she still left it up to me to make it happen.

I took myself to classes and then bought an appointment book when I got sent out on auditions. The bug has to bite you in order for you to have the drive and passion it takes to succeed, even at the teenage level, and that didn't happen to me. I approached auditions the way other kids did their tennis and flute lessons. It was something to do after school.

That cost me when I auditioned for *Foxfire*, a feature being made from the Joyce Carol Oates novel about a secret gang of girls ("Foxfire") who form lasting ties after beating up a teacher who has sexually harassed them. I read for the main character, "Legs" Sadovsky, a complex heroine described as part revolutionary, part Robin Hood, bold, sexy, smart. At the audition, I let my rebellious streak fly. I could not tell whether the casting director was shocked or entertained, but she kept having me return.

It got to the point where after a half dozen callbacks there seemed to be a real possibility that I might get the lead. In fact, as my agent told me, they were considering only one other girl, a teenage actress from Los Angeles named Angelina Jolie. It was an incredible opportunity, yet I thumbed my nose at it, as I did so much of life, by getting high in the waiting room at my final audition.

I cringe when I think of how I must've looked, repeatedly sticking my head in my oversized Betsey Johnson bag and snorting coke. I blew the audition—literally. My mom, acting teacher, and agent consoled me as if I cared. I didn't.

Partying consumed me. A short time after losing the part, I was at a club with a pack that included a cute alternative rocker who was having a moment in the spotlight and the son of another famous rocker who, like me, had always been in the periphery of the spotlight. The alt rocker was also a closet heroin junkie. The celebrity spawn, again like me, was a coke fiend. All of us were out of control—how far out of control was apparent when at about two or three in the morning I went to pee and the cute alt rocker boy stuck his fist in the stall. It was covered with coke.

"Go for it," he cackled.

What was happening? I was in the toilet. This dude was half in the stall with me, offering a fistful of coke. Boundaries were being obliterated. Did they even exist? I didn't know and didn't care. It was about getting high. I leaned forward. Snorted once. Then again.

In the spring, it was déjà vu all over again when my mom received a call from school saying that I'd missed so many days of class that I'd have to repeat tenth grade if I wanted to stay at the Professional Children's School. Since she hadn't been much of a student as a kid and didn't apply any rules as an adult, she didn't get mad as much as she expressed annoyance at the problem it created for her. She had to find a new school for me—and not just any school. I needed one that wouldn't hold me back.

In the meantime, as the school year drew to a close, I had my own personal problems. Much to my dismay, Elle started dating our creepy coke dealer. I advised her against it. I thought he was sleazy and the situation would only lead to trouble, which was what happened. Through the dealer, she began hanging out with another guy, an older dude known for dealing heroin.

I didn't like him. He'd gotten a friend of mine's older sister hooked on smack. I had few limits, but heroin was one of them. That drug scared me. One afternoon, Elle and I were lying on the grass in Central Park when she sat up and looked straight at me from within her deep-set dark eyes.

"I think I want to try it," she said.

I knew she meant heroin. And I knew it was because of the dude she was hanging out with.

"If you do it, I'm not going to talk to you again," I said.

And I didn't. Nearly two months went by before I spent time with Elle again. We crossed paths and arranged to get coffee. I'd missed her. But seeing my friend up close shocked me. During the time I'd avoided her, she'd changed. She had bags under her eyes, her skin was gray, and she'd lost weight. She was dressed up the way we'd always dressed, but something about it didn't look right on her. As we talked, I thought, *Boy, if she looks like that, what the hell do I look like?*

Granted, Elle was doing heroin and I wasn't, but her wasted appearance was one of the few moments up to that point where I paused to step outside myself and look as honestly as possible at my life. Instead of going to a club that night, I stayed home. I remember going into my room and studying myself in the mirror. I looked at my face and eyes close up. I didn't see that same ghost-like pallor that I saw in Elle, but what I did see wasn't good.

My inner voice underscored the point by shouting at me. I had to change before I ended up like Elle.

TWENTY

Dream On

At the end of the year, my mom enrolled me in Beekman, a small high school housed in a brownstone on Fiftieth between Second and Third. With only a couple of hundred students, it offered special attention from grades nine through twelve. I thought of it as a kind of academic halfway house. When they said I wouldn't have to stay back for tenth grade if I attended summer school, I told my mom it was perfect.

On the first day of summer school, I reported to a room where all the summer school students gathered for orientation. A guy that I'd babysat a couple times when we'd first moved to New York saw me come through the door and shouted to the entire room, "Hey, that's Steven Tyler's daughter."

I wanted to turn around and walk out, but I didn't have that option. There was nothing I could do except slink into a desk, cross my arms, look pissed off, and glare at anyone who dared look in my direction. Then, in walked Gillian. Though I didn't dare show my excitement, I brightened inside at the sight of her.

Goldstein! I hadn't seen her for a few months, but I sensed that I'd be seeing a lot more of her.

She sat next to me, and we quickly caught up, cramming

months of news into minutes. We were interrupted by the start of orientation. The two of us traded disinterested looks as the teachers spoke. Halfway through, we left the room and got stoned in a stairwell around the corner from the school. I found out she lived downtown with her parents, whom I met a few days later when I showed up for dinner. They were warm, funny, loving, and involved with each other. I envied their family discussion at the dinner table, their sense of connectedness.

Yet for whatever reasons—maybe it was the artist in her—Gillian's soul was as restless as mine. We became inseparable. In fact, with Elle strung out, I leaned on Gillian all summer.

In the fall, we moved to a larger apartment on Sixty-eighth Street, between Second and Third avenues. My mom made the change after she won an increase in support from my father. He already paid for my school, so the extra money was enough for her to find a larger apartment. When she asked my opinion about it, I expressed ambivalence. As I told her, I planned on moving out when I turned eighteen, which was the following year, so if she wanted to spend two thirds of her monthly income on rent, it was her business; I didn't really care.

At seventeen, I barely hid my disdain for her. We had our good moments, but for the most part, I resented what a lame parent she'd been. Somehow she was able to afford Manolo shoes and hair appointments with Oscar Blandi, and yet she complained constantly about not having any money. One day she came home wearing a new fur hat. When she asked my opinion, I didn't give it good reviews. Unfazed, she looked in the mirror and said, "No, Mia, I look classy."

"Really?"

"Very Madison Avenue."

"If you say so."

"Tallarico!"

Gillian's voice rose from the sidewalk loud and clear, cutting through the noise of the city starting its day. After we moved, every morning began that way: with my friend outside our building, yelling my last name.

As soon as I heard her voice, I hurried downstairs and we walked to school. We made it there by nine a.m. every day except Friday. On Friday, the upper classes, eleventh and twelveth grades, were dismissed at eleven. With little incentive to sit in classes for just two hours, we blew off school in favor of Bloomingdale's and then headed to the Sheep Meadow in the park, where we smoked pot and hung out with skateboarders.

As a result of no longer hanging out with Elle, I did much less coke. I still got high, smoked, and drank, but I felt better, clearer, and less manic. Gillian was a good influence. And so was the boy with whom I fell in love.

His name was Sean, and we met in mid-September at a charity rock show featuring Slash, Billy Idol, and others at Irving Plaza. I'd tagged along with my mom and some of her friends. After finding the VIP room, I asked my mom for a cigarette. A social smoker, she pulled out a box of Dunhills, the expensive British cigarette. I'd forgotten she smoked those. I didn't like them and said no thanks.

I looked around the VIP room, hoping I could spot someone I knew, or someone I wanted to get to know, who might have a real cigarette, and that's when I spotted Sean. He looked like a rocker dude. Skinny. Chin-length hair. Cute. I went up to him and pulled out the line I used on every boy that I liked:

"Can I bum a cigarette?"

I bet that's half the reason any young person smokes. It's social and offers an easy way to meet other people. Sean pulled out a pack and over the course of the concert we hung out together and shared more than a few smokes as we talked. Conversation was easy. We barely paid attention to the music. Before I left, I gave him my phone number. I knew that I liked him in a way that was different from other guys when later that night I lay in bed wondering if he'd call, and when. If he did call, well, I worried what he would think of the way I looked, because my mom and I had had our makeup professionally done before the show and I couldn't re-create the work of a professional makeup artist.

"That's so not like you," Gillian said.

"I know."

"So you like him, don't you?"

I nodded, smiling.

It was the next morning, and I told her everything as soon as I saw her.

"How old is he?"

"Three and a half years older than me."

"He's twenty!"

"Yeah," I said, filling in the other details: he'd grown up in the city with his mom. He was a singer in a band called the Whole Earth Mamas.

"He got that name from watching an interview with my dad," I said. "It's like there's already a connection."

"He's not Puerto Rican?" she asked.

"No," I said.

"Your mom's going to love him."

He called three days later. For our first date, Sean and I and his friend Tim went to a show and then to his place. He shared a stu-dio apartment on Twenty-third and Ninth with a red-haired pub-licist. A spitfire, Nancy was his best friend, but Sean assured me they weren't romantically involved. That was good. But I saw only one bed. My comment elicited a laugh from Sean, who crossed the room and pulled his mattress down from the wall, explaining it was a Murphy bed.

"Cool," I said. "I've never seen one before."

Sean had his own moment of jealousy when, after saying good night, I said that I'd share a cab uptown with his friend Tim. But I gave him the kind of kiss that let him know he need not worry about my newfound affection straying. I wasn't that kind of girl. Nor was he that kind of guy. More important was discovering the wholeness I got from connecting to him in a meaningful way. The interest he took in me—not just physically but in what I thought, the music I liked, the things that were me—let me feel as if I'd found a missing piece of the puzzle that was my life.

Just as Gillian had predicted, my mom approved of Sean. So did my dad, with whom we spent Christmas in Boston. We stayed in a hotel by the water because all of us were going to watch fireworks from the wharf. After checking in, we went for a walk and smoked a joint. We talked about going snowboarding over the coming days, as both of us had recently gotten into the sport. Sean was even wearing his new tinted snowboarding goggles.

When we got back, my dad came into the room to give us his version of the dad talk. Sean was my first real boyfriend, and Dad wanted to check him out more. Sean and I hadn't anticipated that. We were very stoned but trying hard to come off as straight. We had no idea whether we were pulling it off or whether my dad was pretending not to notice, or whether he noticed but didn't want to say anything.

But after my dad left, I looked at Sean and cracked up. I hadn't realized it and my dad hadn't said anything, but my boyfriend of three months had left his snowboarding goggles on the whole time.

"Why'd you do that?" I asked.

"I didn't want him to see my eyes," he said.

"Good thinking," I said. "With those goggles on, that's probably all he looked at."

Sean was good for me. We hung out with friends, went to hip-hop shows, smoked a lot of pot, and partied with friends. On weekends, we played paintball and laser tag. We were always busy. His roommate, Nancy, made sure we were on the guest list of all the good parties, and if she wasn't somehow connected to the event or its promoter, my mom knew everyone else.

It was strange to cross paths with my mom at a party and use that as our time to catch up with each other. But it was a safe milieu of air kisses, hugs, superficial questions, and then the quick "see you later at home." Only I spent more time, at least quality time, at Sean's than I did at my own home. He went to parties because I persuaded him to go out with me, but if given his choice, he preferred to hang out, smoke weed, play video games, and make music with his friends.

On nights we stayed at his place, we ordered in from a Chinese restaurant across the street from his apartment. About six months into being boyfriend-girlfriend, I went through a phase where I cooked and played housewife. I made cookies in the afternoon so that it smelled nice when he came home from band practice. I didn't see it then, but I was desperately looking for family and I was trying to create it with Sean.

Sean was older than me, and the age difference came into play as he was more into hanging out with his friends while I was caught in a difficult netherworld between home and someplace that wasn't home. Although I wouldn't spend the whole night at his place until I'd turned eighteen, his apartment was where I took refuge when things got heated with my mom, and toward the end of 1996 they came to an intense boil.

Don't Want the Pain

The needles left a light black stain on my right arm as the gun went deep into my skin. Gritting my teeth, I watched as a large, intricately rendered tree took shape from a bunch of orange and yellow squiggles the tattoo artist had sketched between my bicep and wrist. The tattoo was even more striking than I'd pictured.

This was the third four-hour session I'd sat through. I'd need dozens more sessions before Kari, the tattoo artist, finished. She stopped for a moment to flex her hand and ask how I was doing.

"OK," I replied, even though both of us knew it hurt so intensely that it put me in a zone where the pain became almost pleasurable.

Of course that was part of the point of tattoos, right? It wasn't just the picture on my skin. It was also the experience of getting it.

Altogether, I have close to two dozen tattoos, and each one reminds me of a story. I can look at one and remember exactly where I was and how I was feeling at that time. I was eighteen years old when I got my first one. I was on vacation in Florida with two friends and I admired a small, tribal-looking tattoo a guy had on his arm. That night, I got an "M" on my lower back. Within a year of that, I got a fairy on the top of my right bicep. It covered scars from when I cut myself.

That one brings back difficult memories. On my right wrist I have two flowers, one on the front, the other on the back. They're gorgeous roses, lavender and red, and they're probably the prettiest of all my tattoos. I never put much thought into the quality of my tattoos and always went to low-end shops until I got the roses, and that was because of their significance.

I got the first one in '05 when I separated from my ex, Dave, and I got the second a year later when our divorce was finalized. They're my freedom flowers.

Getting the tree on my arm was inevitable, I suppose. Starting with my memories of the woods in Sunapee, I've always been fascinated by how the roots of trees grow into the ground, while the rest grows skyward. We see only part of the story. They have mysterious, labyrinthine worlds at both ends. They sway. They make noise in the wind. They seem to have emotions. They're old, timeless, wise, and alive.

My boyfriend, Brian, has a tree, and his inspired me to fill the space on my arm between the fairy and the roses with a large, intricate tree. I've always known I wanted to get a sleeve, my entire arm tattooed, and as I studied Brian's, a tree made sense to me, too. In fact, one afternoon, after we'd talked about it, I happened to see a poster from the movie Pan's Labyrinth, *a picture of trees with gnarled trunks, twisted branches, and a little girl looking up at them. Pictured from behind, she reminded me of a photo my mom took of me when I was little.*

A few days later, I went online and looked at pictures of trees. One caught my attention. It was a tree made out of naked women. I saw the name of the lady credited as the artist and typed her name in MySpace.

"She's got to be on MySpace if she's a tattoo artist," I said.

Sure enough, I found her: Kari Barba. I sent her an e-mail, and then I sent her link to Brian, asking if he knew of her. Brian wrote back, "Have I heard of her? Are you kidding me? She's the number one female tattoo artist in the world."

"How's your hand?" I asked Kari, who'd paused to flex it again.

Petite and super cute, she had a wrist problem that limited the amount of time she was able to work, but I appreciated the vibe of a woman working on me instead of a guy. I told her that I'd never had the fairy on my arm finished because it was awkward having to take down part of my shirt and try to keep my boob covered while fending off the dude's advances.

It had usually been like that in the past. The guy would always find a reason why he couldn't finish and ask if I wanted him to do it at his house that night. No thanks. But Kari was cool and old-school, and I enjoyed everything about my sessions with her—everything, that is, but the pain.

As the tree materialized on my arm in color, complexity, and character, and the little, slightly Goth-looking girl stood in front of it, I wondered how much more tattooing I could stand. After my last session, I'd driven home from her Anaheim shop and realized that I didn't want the pain anymore. I was too far into the tree to stop, but I didn't enjoy it anymore. That was a big epiphany for me. It was like waking up with your dude and realizing you're done with his shit and not going to take it anymore.

The problem was that I still envisioned one more, actually, two more extensive tattoos on my body—specifically on each side of my rib cage. I wanted one of my mom from an old Life magazine photo of her dancing and looking uncharacteristically happy and carefree, a different woman than the one I knew. I wanted the other one to be my dad in his trademark rock star pose, clutching the microphone.

It was really all about the idea of getting my mom tattooed on me. It would, I thought, be fitting if I gave her one last chance to hurt me.

But did I need that? Was I willing to go through more pain on account of her, even if I was the one in control? I mentioned something about it to Kari, who shook her head and said one major project at a time. Then, later, as I talked about it with Brian, I heard myself speaking in that kind of detached way, and something about listening to myself, about looking at myself from a distance, made me pause.

Yes, shit had happened in my life, plenty of shit, and it was my job to deal, not dwell. I needed to heal, not hurt.

As for the tattoos, I had to think about it . . .

Part Three

"I think I should warn you all, when a vampire bites it, it's never a pretty sight. No two blood suckers go out the same way. Some yell and scream, some go quietly, some explode, some implode . . ."

—*Edgar Frog, from* The Lost Boys

TWENTY-ONE

Red Marks

Once I'd turned seventeen, my mom started freaking out about the child support money from my dad that she was going to lose when I turned eighteen and moved out, as I promised every time we got into an argument (and even when we were on good terms). Because she knew that wasn't an idle threat, it sent her into a tailspin, the result of which was a $50,000 deal to write her autobiography, *Dream On: Livin' on the Edge with Steven Tyler and Aerosmith.*

She told me the news about her deal one afternoon as I made a pit stop after school before meeting Gillian and Sean, and then about a week or two later I met her collaborator, a nice guy, I'm sure. I paid them little attention as they worked. My mom poured her energy into that project. It's fascinating to look back and think about the change that came over her when she seemed to have a purpose. I mean, something to do with your life—what a concept!

She focused on the work by taking speed and/or diet pills and drinking. Over time, the pages turned into a booklike pile. One night, she sat down next to me as I watched TV and thrust a handful of pages at me, insisting that I read the latest version of her introduction or a certain part about her parents or some revelation about my dad. It was a scene that was repeated over and over, and each time I refused to read, which pissed her off.

I knew better than to read it. I'd overheard enough conversations between her and her writer or her friends, to whom she either told or relived stories, to be appalled by and scared of her endeavor. On the surface, it was fine. Having lived an interesting life, she had every right to pen a memoir. But what turned me off was her motivation for writing the book. She had in mind a payday, not posterity, and it became obvious she intended to write not the truth but what she thought would sell, which was sex, drugs, and rock and roll—and all at my dad's expense.

Was my dad perfect? An angel? No. By age seventeen, I knew the strengths and shortcomings of both my parents, or at least I had my version of them. One was out of her mind and angry, the other was a narcissistic rock star. Bottom line in terms of my dad: though his work, indeed his art, had taken him on an unusual course in life, he was a good, loving man. I resented the hell out of my mom for trying to make a buck by portraying him in another light.

Though she knew how I felt, one day she thrust the prologue at me when I came home from school, demanding that I read it. I saw the title, "Diving for Diamonds," and rolled my eyes. I asked if I had to read it. My mom said yes. It was about a trip she and my dad took to Hawaii. She walked by a jewelry store and admired a diamond bracelet. As I turned the pages, I guessed what was coming and said, "I don't want to read any more."

"Why?" she replied. "It's true."

That didn't necessarily mean she should tell her child—or the world. But she pushed me to continue. Long story short, she wrote that my dad had bought the bracelet, put it around his junk, and told her to go diving.

I threw the pages at her, repulsed. I told her that I didn't want to read any more of her book. Ever!

"Why?" she said defiantly. "It's your life."

"No, it's not my life. It's *your* fucked-up life. I don't want any-thing to do with it. I don't even think you should write this book."

Looking back, I'm not sure if she wanted my opinion, my contri-butions, or if she wanted me to read her book as a way of justifying her take on the issues that shaped her life, and my life, too—issues that we'd argued over for years. I doubt she was reaching out to me. The book turned me off to her even further.

Angry and disgusted, I dug in my heels and took a serious stand against her. One day I yelled at her to get a job, not attack my dad.

"This is my version of my life," she argued.

"It's all negative," I said. "You aren't going to make the world hate Dad the way you do no matter how hard you try. People love him."

She didn't get it. Though she tried to cover it with makeup, great hair, designer labels, and a conspicuous perch at hot parties, she had a blind spot: her own woe-is-me self. I didn't know whether to laugh or cry when I looked around at the apartment and saw stacks of diet and self-help books she'd bought over the years and never read. If she read them, she never put the things she learned into practice. She gained weight. She burned through friends. If things are so bad that you complain all the time, why not do something about it?

Living as the anti–Gilmore Girls had a deleterious effect on nearly every aspect of my life. I disconnected from school, where I cut classes as if I had a blanket exemption. Toward the end of the school year, I received a progress report—or lack-of-progress report—saying that I was getting a D in one of my classes. My teacher played in a band. In an attempt to up my grade, I went to see him play at a club. I got drunk with him, and we made out. I still got a D.

I vented to Sean, though that makes me sound more mature

than I was. Most of the time, I was angry, frustrated, and a handful to be with. I also let my dad know that I was fed up with my mother and didn't want to live with her anymore. Then Beekman said they didn't want me back for twelfth grade. I'd missed too much school. I begged my dad to let me move in with him. I sounded like I did when I had the same conversations with him as a little girl. Nothing had changed; things were only more complicated. I sounded like a broken record: everything was fucked.

I think my dad felt genuinely bad for me and wanted to help within the limitations of his life and career. He came through town several times and took me out to eat and shop. It was nice, but the effect was like a Band-Aid on a chest wound. I wanted him to take me away; he couldn't. He suggested boarding school, which seemed like a good idea. My mom and dad and I made several trips together to see various schools outside the New York metropolitan area. It was not fun being cooped up in a car with them. There was too much tension. My mom preceded each trip by reminding me that if I left home my dad would cut off her child support.

One day we were at a school in New Jersey. I barely uttered a word as we toured the grounds. Then I went into the admissions office for an interview. A well-dressed woman about my mom's age sat across from me and asked what I liked to read and study. I'll never forget what happened next; after I offered several short, obviously unsatisfying (and perhaps troubling) answers, she stared at me as if she were trying to see inside me. It was a look of intensity concealed by kindness. Finally, she asked me to name one thing I liked about myself.

I shut my eyes and took a deep breath. Then I looked at the window before facing the lady again.

"I don't know," I said. "I can't think of anything."

My mom described her book as a cathartic experience, one that had forced her in a helpful way to face a past that she had determined to forget. But one day, after the proofs came in, I looked at the first page and saw that in chapter one she wrote, "My real name is Kathleen Victoria, and I'm not going to give my last name because I want to leave my father out of this." You didn't need Freud to deduce that she was still in denial.

Many years had to pass before I was able to understand her better and grasp the pain she was in, since she'd totally desensitized me to her plight. But I remember coming home one night and noticing a strange mark on her arm. She was seated in a chair in the living room, coffee and cigarettes nearby. Telling me how she'd been correcting the proofs on her book, she did that thing where she wanted me to see her arm but pretended she didn't want me to.

"What's that on your arm?" I asked.

"What?" she said, glancing at the mark on her arm and pushing her sleeve over it. "Nothing."

Over the next week I noticed that and another mark. Two of them. Red and raw. Finally, one day, I grabbed her arm and stared at the red mark.

"What the fuck are these?" I asked.

Reluctantly, she revealed that she used to burn herself with cigarettes in high school and had done it again recently in her bedroom as she relived those painful years for her book. I stood in front of her, looking at her arm; I was confused at first, and then I felt a burning anger toward her. It was a moment that should've drawn me to her. On *Gilmore Girls,* it would've been an emotional turning point for the mother and daughter. But to me, it seemed like one more piece of evidence that my mom was a mess.

Why the fuck would she do that to herself? Even with all the drugs I'd smoked, snorted, and swallowed, I'd never thought about hurting myself.

"Don't you think that's fucked up?" I asked Sean later, as I recounted what my mom had done to herself.

"Totally," he said.

It's interesting. Not much more was ever said on the subject.

Not between me and my mom or me and Sean or Gillian or any of the others I may have confided in. Yet through all the dope smoking, video game playing, and shit that I did, I would find myself occasionally thinking about those marks on her arm, and wondering—no, asking myself—Why?

TWENTY-TWO

City Ass

In the fall, I enrolled at Robert Louis Stevenson School on West Seventy-fourth Street, a small school that touted itself as a therapeutic environment for "bright underachieving adolescents" challenged by a range of difficulties from depression to attention deficit disorder to plain old trouble getting along.

In theory, it was a perfect choice for me. In practice, I was too undisciplined and unfocused to care about this or any other school. I hated my mother—and my life. I remember telling people that I was depressed, but in retrospect it wasn't accurate. Because I wasn't depressed, not in the way people battle depression. I was lost, unmoored, drifting without a port, anchor, or destination.

In search of excuses to miss school, I went on dozens of auditions. Despite callbacks, I was repeatedly turned down. I knew you weren't supposed to take those rejections personally, but I did. My outlook was straight out of the movie *Reality Bites*, when Ethan Hawke's character says, "There's no point to any of this. It's all just a . . . a random lottery of meaningless tragedy and a series of near escapes."

Pointlessness. I suffered that in spades. And pain—the kind

that makes you groan and sigh and walk around wearing a weary glaze. If not weary, I had a full complement of expressions hanging in my closet, including disinterested, blasé, and burned out. It's fair to wonder how someone with so much going for her, so many advantages, could be in so much pain. The answer is simple. Like anyone else, I needed the things money couldn't buy.

One day I walked into an assembly and nearly crashed into my old therapist. She was the school's counselor. Oh my God. It wasn't pleasant. She immediately whispered to the school's principal to keep a close eye on me. And she did. About a month later, I came to school with bloodshot eyes. She yanked me into her office, thinking I'd been smoking pot.

I hadn't been. It was eight in the morning and I'd been up all night. I was tired. I told her as much and said she should be paying attention to the kids snorting E in the bathrooms and leave me alone. All I needed was sleep.

I tried to cover up my feelings by hanging with Sean, who was more into getting high and playing video games with his friends than listening to my broken record of complaints. Gillian was living with a shit-bag boyfriend. That left me feeling alone and trapped by my thoughts and emotions. One night that fall—I remember it was fall because I was anticipating my eighteenth birthday and finally moving away from my mother, whose existence, sadly, had for me become the personification of scratching fingernails on a chalkboard—I felt like all of my pent-up frustration was going to cause me to explode if I didn't do something.

I was in my bedroom and staring at the walls, when I picked up my Chanel compact (the one with four shades of eye shadow inside) and began to scratch my arm with it. I started doing it absentmindedly, not even aware until it started to hurt.

Then, for some reason, the pain registered with me in a different way. It hurt so good. I paused and recalled the red marks on my mother's arm. "I used to burn myself with cigarettes when I was a teenager," she'd said. I looked at the compact in my hand and the red marks on my arm. The next time I pressed the sharp edge of the compact against my skin, scratching harder and harder, until the red mark on my arm opened up and I saw blood.

As I cut myself, I didn't realize that I was crying. Once I saw blood, I stopped. It was as if I woke up. I felt a small sense of relief, something between a head rush and a giant exhalation of breath. I remember sitting in my room as if in a daze, knowing I'd just done something simultaneously terrible and remarkable. It was also intimate and private. I knew that I wouldn't tell anyone. I also knew that I'd do it again.

In December, I turned eighteen and obsessed about my exodus from home. The following month my mom's book was published. She received mixed if not poor reviews from those who took notice of it in the first place. I felt a measure of vindication at seeing it fail. I nearly gagged when I saw that one of the last chapters was titled "Mia's Sister, the Movie Star." I never spoke about it with Liv. I didn't want to.

By the time she'd finished promoting the book, I was living at Sean's on a mostly full-time basis. After his publicist roommate moved to Los Angeles, I settled into his place. I'd been bringing my stuff over in small portions for months, so it wasn't a big deal. I didn't have an official good-bye with my mom. At night, I'd call and either tell her or leave a message that I wasn't going to be home. Now that I was eighteen, there was little she could do about it.

But moving in with Sean failed to solve my problems in the way that I'd imagined. Neither he nor anyone else knew that I had become a cutter. Not only that, I had graduated from my compact to one of the small knives that I collected. I didn't do it often, just when I felt overwhelmed and needed to exert, or at least try to exert, control and find relief.

The cutting added a layer of taboo, shame, and secrecy. Then I started to hate Sean's apartment. It was small, and he always had friends over because he was the only one in his group who lived on his own. The situation made me claustrophobic. I didn't feel comfortable there and that exacerbated a greater problem, namely that I didn't feel like there was anyplace for me . . . anywhere.

That's what made it so ironic when I landed a part on *Michael Hayes*, a gritty cop series starring David Caruso. On my first day of work, I showed up and was directed to a large motor home, a "honey wagon," that was my dressing room. The PA who showed me to it pointed out that my name was on the door.

"That's your place," he said, blowing hot air on his cold hands but still smiling. "Home sweet home."

I'd been tired of auditioning when my agent persuaded me to do just one more. The last one to read that day for the casting director, I went in with the worst attitude. Like: *I know you're going to reject me, but what the fuck, I'm here anyway.* Then I left for another audition my mom's friend had set up for me. That one was for a new morning talk show with four hosts and Barbara Walters. It was called *The View*.

As I waited for my meeting at *The View*, my agent called with news that I'd got the part on *Michael Hayes*. I was so happy. I jumped up and down in the waiting room. Although *The View* was looking for a young cohost, I was, at eighteen, too young and too uninformed to sit in on a daily news-driven show. The demands would've been more than I could've handled at the time.

But *Michael Hayes* was right up my alley. It was shot over a few days on location in a cemetery. It was cold out. I drank cup after cup of coffee to warm up and in the process got totally wired on caffeine. After the last night of shooting, my friend John Bogush and I went to dinner at this Upper East Side joint called the Velvet Room. We liked it because it was super dark, lit only by candles.

Everyone has one of those people whom they look back on as epitomizing the best times, and Bogush was that person for me. I met him at camp when I was fourteen, and we were always friends after that. My mom loved him. They had the same birthday. He was like my older brother. He opened doors for me. If we were drinking, he made sure I got home. We used to walk through the Museum of Natural History or visit his friend Quincy at Juilliard.

There weren't enough of those good times with Bogush. That spring, I dropped out of Robert Louis Stevenson. Although I was a mere one language credit short of being able to graduate, school was more than I could handle. It was symptomatic of everything else. I also got sick of Sean and had one of those "this isn't working" kind of talks on the phone. In slacker fashion, we continued to see each other for another six years, but without the boyfriend-girlfriend commitment.

Beach Boy Brian Wilson once wrote a song about feeling like a cork floating on the ocean, and I felt similarly but with different references. I was a whisper in the din of the city. After Sean's, I bounced from friend to friend, landing for the longest stretch on the sofa of Sean's friend Dan. Dan and his girlfriend, Karen, lived near South Street Seaport. I probably would've slept on the streets without their generosity. I didn't want to go back home with my mom.

That summer I put myself into a New York City community high school to graduate. My parents were pleased. Maybe they would've felt differently if they'd known what the school was really like. Everyone referred to it as "City Ass." The name fit it. It was the asshole of public education. In general, no one—not the students or the teachers—cared enough. Most of the girls in my class had at least one child. But there were exceptions. One girl who I adored had a three-year-old and a one-year-old. She was sixteen. She was determined to go to college.

It was years later that I appreciated the few like her that I met for providing me with the best lessons I ever learned in school. They'd had every bad break in life or made every bad mistake, yet they were past making excuses and blaming other people. They got their ass to school, sat in classes, and did their work.

• • •

> They had to create themselves because no one was going to do it for them. They knew what I still had to learn.

After sleeping on Dan and Karen's sofa, I moved in with another of Sean's friends, a girl named Taylor, who lived in Queens and offered me her couch because I was, quite frankly, out of options if I didn't want to go back home. I was lucky she had an empty sofa and an understanding roommate. Ricky, her roommate, was the first Jehovah's Witness I'd met. He was hipper than I expected from a guy who spent much of his free time handing out Witness literature.

But I was willing to have my horizons expanded. I wasn't in a position where I could indulge in prejudices or preconceptions. Nor was it my nature to. From the time I met Ricky, those who hung out with him and Taylor made fun of him for having a small wiener, and that made me curious as all hell.

"How small is it?" I asked Taylor one day.

She didn't know.

"Then how does everyone know it's small?" I asked.

She didn't know that either.

That's when I started asking Ricky to show it to me. For a day or two I said it as a tease. I didn't realize how serious or perhaps curious I was until I began trying to seduce him. I don't know why it was important to me. But my slight thirst turned into the worst case of dry-mouth ever known. Finally, one night when we were alone, after we'd been drinking and I was telling him how good the sex would be, he let me lock his bedroom door.

"Lights on or off?" he asked.

"Let's start with them on," I said.

Though I tried to be sensitive, there was no hiding my true intent. It was like an unveiling. As his boxers slid down, I had to keep from exclaiming "Oh my God." To his credit, he let me measure it against my thumb. But his eyes begged my opinion with a vulnerability I'd never encountered before in a boy.

"How is it?" he asked.

"Looks good," I said. "Let's see if it works."

We continued to sleep together, though I can't say I enjoyed the physical part after that first encounter. His thingie aside, I simply wasn't attracted to Ricky. There wasn't any chemistry. But I needed a place to stay. Not that I slept in. The truth was, I couldn't wait to get out of bed. I rose early in the morning, showered, dressed, got on the subway, and went to work.

Through City Ass, I'd gotten an internship with a casting agency on Twentieth Street. I usually arrived around eight. Since that was about two hours before the casting agency opened, I sat in a coffee shop, usually in a booth, paging through the newspaper and staring out the window, until I saw someone open up the agency.

It was a dismal way to start the day, and while sitting there one morning I flashed back with bittersweet recognition to an afternoon in Sunapee. I was ten years old and parked in front of the TV, watching Sally Jessy Raphael. The bespectacled queen of daytime talk was interviewing an expert about teenagers. I was too young to understand the nuances, but at the time all I wanted was to be a teenager, and Sally Jessy's expert stated that the pre-teen years began at ten years old.

I jumped up. I was ten! I found my mom and excitedly told her the news. *Guess what! Guess what! I'm almost a teenager.* After listening to my explanation, she put her hands on my shoulders and told me not to be in such a hurry to grow up. I looked at her as if she'd come down a mountain speaking a language I didn't understand.

"What I mean is be careful what you wish for," she said.

Why on earth those words had hammered themselves back into my consciousness at that moment was one of those things that make you sit up straight and acknowledge the pure and occasional freakiness of the human brain. It was proof the CPU was at work even as I sat in a semi-stuporous fog left over from the previous evening. I understood the frightening message that had ridden a magic carpet of caffeine through the thickets of dulled synapses in my head.

I didn't have to look far. It was right in front of me—my reflection in the coffee shop window, giving me a knowing stare. I'd counted the days until I turned eighteen and could live on my own. And now? Well past that magic milestone, I was sleeping with a guy so I could have a place to stay, cutting myself in private to relieve the pain, and working a crap job to have a place to go and something to do during the day.

Be careful what you wish for. *In-fucking-deed.*

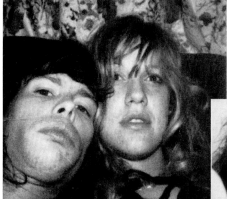

My mom and dad a month before
I was born.

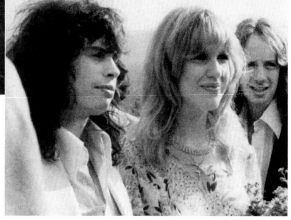

My parents' half-hippie,
half-traditional wedding.

Me at two days old.

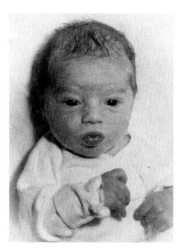

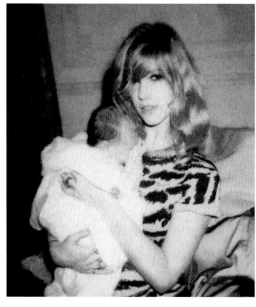

Mom and me (I was a few
months old in this photo).

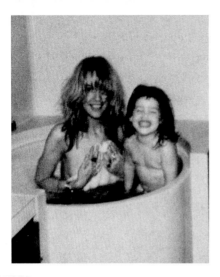

My mom and me playing around in the tub at our Fort Lauderdale house.

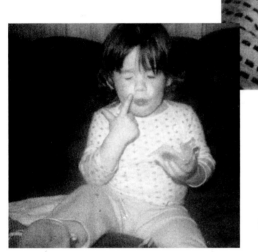

My dad and me asleep in the same position.

Here's me at two years old, doing my best Bobbi Brown impression after getting into my mom's cosmetic bag.

Me in my pink tutu at two years old. This was before I knew I was a black tights kind of girl.

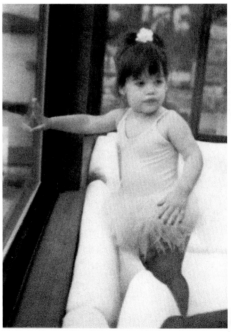

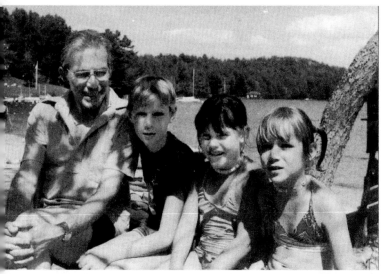

Papa Vic (my dad's dad), my cousin Darren, me, and my cousin Julia at Dewey Beach in Sunapee.

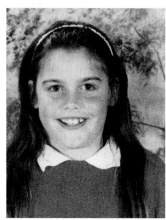

My third-grade class photo.

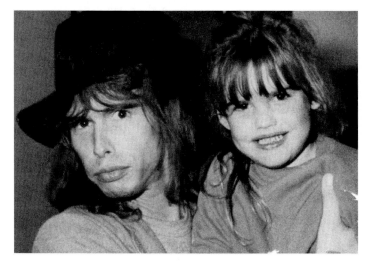

Me and Dad.

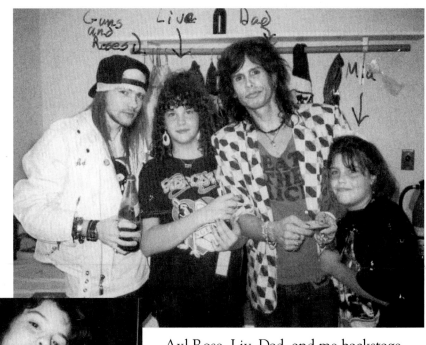

Axl Rose, Liv, Dad, and me backstage at an Aerosmith show in Maine. That was the night I met Liv for the first time. *(Photo: Bebe Buell)*

Liv and me (and our eighties perms).

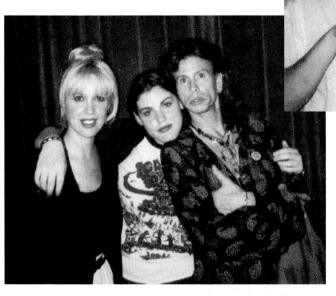

My mom and me at Stagedoor Manor camp.

Mom and Dad at my high school play.

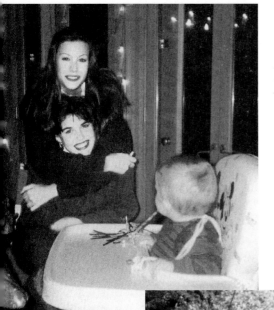

Liv and me in New Hampshire
for my birthday.

Me, Taj, Dad, Chelsea, and Liv
having a picnic in Central Park
in 1993.

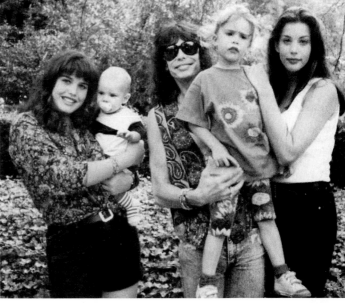

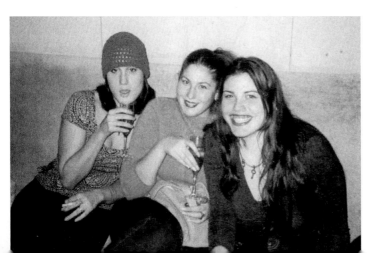

Gillian, her sister
Josie, and me in
New York City
in 2001.

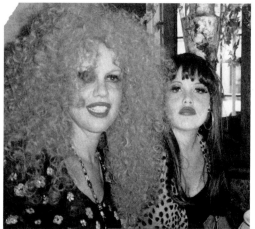

My mom and I are dolled up for Wigstock 1995.

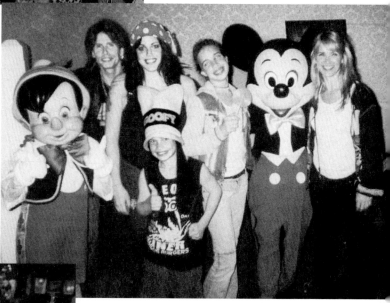

The Tallarico clan at Disneyland in 2002.

A warm moment with Dad.

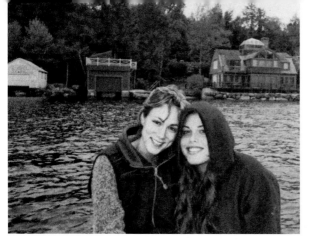

Julia and me on a boat in front of
the house where I grew up. This was
taken right after my mom passed.

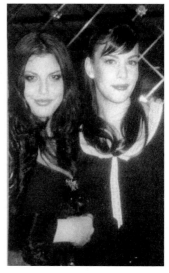

Liv and me at the first
Lord of the Rings pre-
miere. (*Photo: Bebe
Buell*)

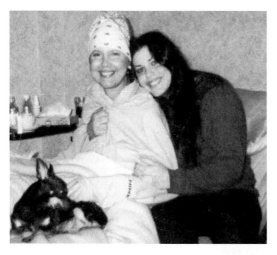

My mom and me at her
hotel when she was sick.

Keith Waa, my mom,
and me.

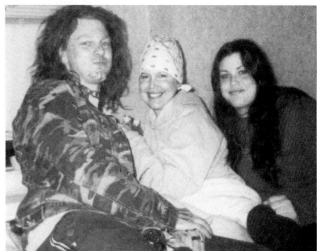

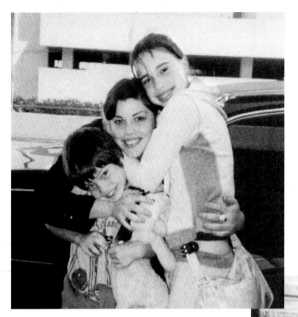

Taj, Chelsea, and me at the airport the day after the MTV Icon concert.

My dad and me in a Massachusetts train station after a visit.

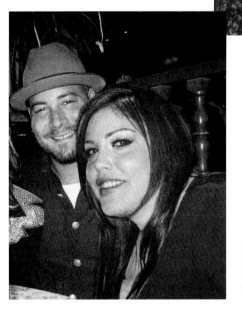

Me and my fiancé, Brian, at a party for a family friend.

TWENTY-THREE

Help, I'm Going Crazy

I reached a point of desperation where I called my dad and told him everything in a tear-filled confession. He rented me a small apartment on Twenty-second and Park, a block and a half from the casting agency. It was the first place we saw (impatient, I just wanted to get something); the top floor was at street level and included a kitchen and living room, and the bedroom was down a short flight of stairs.

I moved in with a mattress and a coffeemaker. Through resourcefulness, I found a couch and a coffee table. I took an old TV from my mom's apartment. Pissed off, my mom refused to have anything to do with a place my dad got me. After I'd been there a few days, my stepmom Teresa and her twin sister came into town and took me shopping at Bed Bath and Beyond. It was as if my dad called in the cavalry. The two of them filled seven shopping carts and settled me in.

I refer to that place as "the devil's apartment" because over the next six months I went crazy. When my internship with the casting agency ended, I didn't have the resources or wherewithal to get another job. I had nothing but time. It piled up the way Crazy

Wally had crammed his little house with junk. Instead of clocks, newspapers, and crap, I had stacks of hours and days.

Once again, I was floating, empty and lost, without any connection to anything or anyone, like an astronaut on a spacewalk without a lifeline. Despite regular check-ins with my parents and outings with friends, in my head I circumnavigated Manhattan in near-total alienation. One night I had dinner with Gillian and some other friends. I had on a long-sleeved shirt to hide the marks from several recent episodes with my knife. Late in the evening, after getting wasted, we were walking through the Village and I pushed up my sleeves without realizing what I was exposing. Gillian immediately noticed and grabbed my arm.

"What's that?" she said. "What're those cuts?"

I reacted exactly as my mom had reacted when I noticed the red marks on her arm. I jerked my arm from her, pushed my sleeves down, and said they were nothing. Gillian yelled at me. I screamed something back, then cried.

In the midst of that animated exchange, a cop car pulled up alongside us. An officer leaned out the passenger window and asked why we were yelling. Just girl stuff, we said. They drove off. But that snapped us back to reality.

"Tallarico," she said, "just tell me, are you doing that to yourself?"

I shook my head.

"I don't want to talk about it."

I didn't want to talk about anything relating to me. During a daytime stopover at my mom's apartment, I took several bottles of her prescription diet pills. She'd taken them for years. The dosage was six per day, but I took six every couple of hours. Soon I began drinking tequila at night to take the edge off of the speed, and then I started to mix the two throughout the day. Compared to a drink like vodka and Red Bull, I was ingesting rocket fuel. I was so loaded that someone should've slapped a sign on my ass: DANGER: COMBUSTIBLE.

I reconnected with Elle, who brought her toxicity back into my life. We went back to our old ways of snorting all of Manhattan. I subsisted on melba toast, cottage cheese, cocaine, tequila, and diet pills. Needless to say, I got frighteningly skinny. I also became paranoid. I refused to go outside if it was light. I stayed in my subterranean bedroom, watching TV into the night, until I heard the prelude to the local news: "It's ten p.m. Do you know where your children are?"

I treated my body as recklessly as every other aspect of my life. I picked up guys at clubs and amused myself by using a glow-in-the-dark ink pen to make notches on my bedroom wall. When the lights were off, my eyes would inevitably search out those marks standing out like a small army of stick figures marching past my bed, and past my lonely heart. I wasn't making love. I was marking time.

Then the accidents began. One time Elle and I did nearly fourteen grams of coke in twelve hours. In my delirium, my nose bled and I ate the stream of bloody mucus. Another time I took twenty hits of E and thought ghosts were walking through me. I developed tremors from the pills. My body was pushing back, fighting for survival.

I couldn't get high enough. I had no idea anymore how high was high. A couple of times I called my dad in a panic that I might have done too much of whatever drug I was doing at the time. But one night was worse than all the others. Alone, I was sitting on my bedroom floor after doing too much blow. With a bottle of tequila parked next to me, I spent God knows how long rocking back and forth in a fit of uncontrollable anxiety. I felt as if all the nervous energy in the world had been injected into my veins.

I didn't have a clue what time it was, but I picked up the phone and called my dad. He picked up right away, so it must've been an odd hour. As soon as I heard his voice, I broke down.

"Help, I'm going crazy," I said.

"Mia, what's wrong, baby?"

"I'm going crazy."

"Slow down. Tell me what's going on."

"People are looking at me," I cried. "I can't go outside. I can't go anywhere . . ."

Calm, my dad turned into a clinician, asking a series of questions that gave him a good idea of the details and gravity of the situation. This was the first time I'd been 100 percent frank with him after one of my emergency calls. I gave him as much information as I had, trying hard to remember as many details as possible, if only to prove to myself that I still had some control over my mind.

"I'm so glad I never did heroin," I said for no reason, other than I was probably thinking of Elle and/or genuinely grateful I hadn't done harder drugs because I had little doubt I'd be dead.

"I'm glad, too, baby," my dad said. "Everything's going to be okay."

He stayed on the phone with me for a while. I was comforted and reassured by his voice, by his presence in my life. Even if it was by phone, he was there for me when I needed him, and he knew what to say and do.

"I'm so sorry," I cried. "I'm insane. I hate this."

Once he felt the immediate crisis had been averted, he told me that he wanted to make some calls to get help. He said that he'd call right back.

"Please," I said.

A short time later, my dad called back. He said that he was sending me to a spa in Malibu for a month, starting the next day. He said everything was arranged, including the car that would pick me up in front of my apartment. He gave me all the necessary information and had me read it back to him. All of a sudden it paid to have a rock star for a dad. He knew exactly what to do in the event of a drug-induced freak-out. As he said, he'd been through it himself.

At noon the next day, I was in the American Airlines terminal at JFK International Airport. On the way there, I'd smoked a
monster joint, a five-paper godfather. I got on the plane and sat in
first class. For the duration of the five-hour flight, I drank Malibu
rum and OJ and mulled which treatments I wanted when I got to
the spa. I looked forward to leaving New York, resting, and feeling
healthier.

TWENTY-FOUR

Promises

A man named Steven met me at the airport. Recognizing me as I came off the plane, he reintroduced himself as a friend of my father's, threw me in his BMW, and drove me to Malibu. He reminded me that he'd helped get my dad sober in the '80s. Ah, the memory came back. I smiled.

"Oh, so that's what's going on," I said.

Steven wore a suit, smelled nice, and from what I remembered he had a big heart. Although he knew that I was blasted, he didn't say anything to that effect. He was probably used to picking up doped-up rock stars. He explained that he was taking me to Promises, a well-known rehab facility in the Malibu hills.

"My dad said it was a spa."

"I told him to say that to you in case you resisted," he said.

"No, I'm cool," I said, lying.

Steven probably knew that, too. He let me melt into the front seat of his car and stare silently out at the new scenery from my tired, bloodshot eyes. I hadn't been to L.A. for years, and everything looked new to me. Even through my sunglasses, the afternoon sun was bright and strong. Steven sped up the 405 freeway, then turned off on the Pacific Coast Highway and drove along the coast. I enjoyed the sight of the ocean shimmering in the distance. I rolled down the window and breathed in the cool air.

"Big difference from New York," Steven said.

"Yeah," I replied. "It's a change."

As Steven led me into the Mediterranean-style mansion that had been transformed into Promises, he finished telling me some of his own background as a former Ivy League graduate who'd been working as a nurse in L.A. while addicted to cocaine, pills, and alcohol. After a four-day binge much like mine left him tweaking in his apartment, his best friend intervened and took him to a twelve-step meeting. That began his recovery. He'd been sober for nearly sixteen years.

I arrived on a Sunday, a free day for those in the residential treatment facility. Walking in, I saw the star of a top TV sitcom barbecuing and a young movie star cooling off in the pool. An attendant showed me to my room. I checked him out; tall, muscled, he was pretty decent looking. I was obsessing about his physical attributes when I realized he was going through my bags. I reached for my stuff.

"What are you doing?" I said.

"It's routine," he said calmly.

"Not for me. Why are you going through my bags?"

"Drugs," he said. "Other stuff on the list of prohibited items. Do you want me to go through the list?"

"No, that's all right."

I was embarrassed as he pulled out a box of tampons. I protested when he took away my nail polish, shampoo, cell phone, and Walkman. But I had nothing to say when he pulled out a small box that I'd stuck in my bag before leaving home.

"What are these?" he said, shaking the box.

"Pills," I said.

"What kind?"

"Diet pills."

"This is why we go through your bags," he said.

• • •

I spent the first week detoxing, a miserable seven days of aches and pains as my brain and body went to war, my body screaming for drugs and my brain saying no, no, no. The severity of one's detox depends on their addiction. Oxycontin is different (and worse) than cocaine, which is different than heroin, and so on. Some people endure tremors and nausea, others struggle with hallucinations and such severe pain they're tranquilized so they don't hurt themselves.

Mine was comparatively mild. Basically, aside from meals and some meetings, I slept for a week as the mix of stimulants and depressants I'd consumed in New York worked its way out of my system. Someone once asked me what the start of treatment was like. I didn't know. Even though I was in it, I was out of it.

But I was still told the rules, and as I came out of my stupor I learned the ropes as well. In addition to living in a completely drug- and alcohol-free environment, treatment consisted of attending daily therapy sessions and twelve-step groups. They enrolled me in what I imagined was every group on the menu: MA (Marijuana Anonymous), CA (Cocaine Anonymous), NA (Narcotics Anonymous), AA (Alcoholics Anonymous), and SLAA (Sex and Love Addicts Anonymous). They also asked me to go to OA (Overeaters Anonymous), but I objected, explaining that despite the diet pills, I was not anorexic, bulimic, or overweight. I was bone thin because of the speed and coke I was doing, not because I cared about being thin. I didn't have an issue with food or my body. Not knowing me, they were reluctant to believe me.

"Guys, I've got every color chip in the rainbow," I said. "I'm just trying to deal with one thing at a time."

My biggest challenge at Promises was privacy. After detoxing, I was given a roommate. It was a space issue. My room was a double, and it had the only empty bed left in the facility. So one afternoon, as I rested between groups and lunch, Lois arrived. She was in her mid-fifties and messed up. She wore jeans, a faded T-shirt, and a threadbare flannel shirt. She looked like a little old man, with a bright red nose and stringy black and gray hair that hit her shoulders unevenly. I guess she had the DTs. She shook, cried, and freaked me out.

"I have to get out of here," I said to one of the attendants.

"That's not going to happen," he said. "Everyone shares a room. No one gets special treatment."

"I'm not asking for special treatment. I'm just bothered by what I see."

"Use it as a part of your treatment. Think about what you saw in yourself. She's not going through anything you didn't."

"I wasn't that bad."

"How do you know?"

"I know," I insisted.

"If you knew so much," he said, "you wouldn't be here."

Touché. But as my head cleared and I began therapy and group sessions, I knew without a doubt that I wasn't an addict. I also knew that was something every other addict said, too. Rehab was the first time in my life that I'd stopped to look honestly and deeply at myself. The therapy I'd had as a child had been about satisfying my mom, and one of the insights I had early in my post-detox therapy and meetings was confirmation that my problems related to my family.

I remember sharing in one of my groups that I didn't feel the need to do drugs as much as I'd been determined to find a way to escape my mom. Almost immediately someone had challenged me, saying, "Bullshit!"

I glared at the guy.

"You don't know my mother," I said.

"You don't know mine," he replied, and then added, "Maybe if both of our mothers had been in therapy as younger women, neither of us would be here."

I smiled. "Yeah. Good point."

Many good points were made in those sessions. For me, Promises was a lifesaver if for no other reason than being there forced a dramatic change in the habits that were driving me insane and got me out of the toxic environment of home. But there was more.

Listening to and interacting with others in groups in their various stages of recovery opened my eyes to the necessity of inner strength and self-reliance. Things I didn't get then came to me years later as the basis of my philosophy of knowing the pain of the tough times will be the source of wisdom and strength later on.

Days at Promises were all about routine. There were meetings, therapy sessions, a brief pause to watch the sun slip down the backside of the Pacific, then reading and chores. The routine was crucial to the regrounding effort. Only the chores changed. One week I was assigned to clean the living room area, another week I had responsibility for the bathrooms, and then another week I shared kitchen duty with a sitcom star who I taught how to eat edamame.

"Are these cooked?" he asked.

"They're cooked, salted, and chilled," I said. "You squeeze 'em right into your mouth." I laughed, hoping he wouldn't go for the obvious dirty joke. "Don't you know anything?"

"Not enough," he said, and then, with a shrug, added, "Look where I am."

Those sorts of comments were plentiful and frequent. I'd be lying if I didn't admit I did my share of eye-rolling and tuning out while in various groups and walking around the facility. You don't go from being fucked up to enlightened in twenty-eight days simply by sitting in twelve-step groups and talking about the people you hurt and the things you screwed up because you got high.

But I clicked with my therapist, a smart, strong, inquisitive woman in her forties. The work we did was slow and painful, as I was wary, cynical, wounded, and distrustful. But she also was patient and skilled at breaking down my barriers. I surprised myself by talking about things I'd kept inside or repressed since they'd happened. I'd never talked about these things before, yet I needed to—and they flooded out.

A few weeks into the process an unexpected thing happened. After our sessions, I found myself bursting into tears for no apparent reason. It was like this surge of emotion and water that had to get out of me. The first time it happened as I rested in the afternoon. I thought things were okay; then, *kaboom!* Another time the dam burst in the middle of dinner. It also happened at night as I tried to read in my bedroom. The next thing I knew I was sobbing.

"I went in the closet, curled up, and cried like a baby," I told my therapist.

"Why the closet?" she asked.

"It's what I used to do when I was a little kid in Sunapee," I said. "When something upset me, I hid in my closet and cried."

She explained that I was reverting back to being six years old, the age when the bad stuff in my life began to happen, when my mom began neglecting me, when I had the hazy impression of having been abused by my babysitter's boyfriend, when I stopped getting the right kind of emotional nourishment and attention.

"This happens when you're going through therapy," she said.

"Make it stop," I said pleadingly.

"You don't want it to stop," she said. "You want to embrace that little girl. You want to understand her. You want to—"

"Why?" I interrupted.

"Have you heard people talk about their inner child?"

"Yes."

"Your inner little girl was hurt when you were younger. You thought you could protect her by shutting her in the closet where no one could find her and hear her crying. But in doing so, you never dealt with that pain. Consequently, that little girl's wounds are as raw and ripe today as they were thirteen years ago. When she hurts, you hurt—even today. You try ignoring her by drinking or using drugs. But, as you found out, that way doesn't work. The only way to get better is to stop sheltering her. Embrace her. Listen to her. Help her understand that what happened won't happen again."

"Why won't it happen again?"

"Because you won't let it. You're older now. You're stronger and smarter. And hopefully you can see that you have a choice.

You can choose to do nothing and continue as you were before you came here. But then you don't grow. You can't realize your potential. You remain stuck in the past."

I nodded.

"Or you can acknowledge that what happened to that little girl was bad and painful and wrong, and then move on with your life," she continued. "I'm not saying to forget it happened. You can't ever do that. But don't dwell. Don't let it hurt you forever. In fact, use it to make you stronger."

I gazed out at the light blue sky and listened to the loud caws of several hungry gulls. She made sense. I got it. But it started sounding like a lecture, and it was too much information. I felt swamped. I rolled my eyes.

"Easier said than done."

"I didn't say it was easy," she said.

TWENTY-FIVE

V-Girl

After a month, I had the option of leaving Promises. Though I was determined to go home, Steven, my therapist, and the staff advised against it. I felt like they were being overly cautious because of their relationship with my father. I argued that I'd acquired the tools and insight I needed to return to my life stronger, healthier, and unlikely to nose-dive into the same self-destructive abyss.

There was a conference call with my dad, Teresa, my therapists, and me on the line at the same time. (My mom wasn't included; with my dad's experience in rehab, she left this to him.) If I chose to leave, they recommended my going to a halfway house. I strongly disagreed.

"My problem isn't drug addiction or alcoholism," I said. "It's the mental shit with my mom, my family, and me trying to figure myself out."

Though they didn't argue, Steven still made a pitch for the halfway house. Then my dad chimed in. Everyone had something to say. To me, they were trying out their version of tough love. But tough love doesn't work on me. The harder they pushed, the more

I resisted. Everyone made good points. In the end, not wanting to disappoint them or cheat myself, I stayed at Promises for another three weeks.

Whatever disappointment I expressed over the extension of my stay was softened by something I kept to myself. Earlier in the day, I'd spied a cute boy checking in. The second I saw him I thought, *Damn, I wish I could hang around for a while longer.* A day or two later, I made it a point to meet him. We spoke by the pool and then again after dinner. He was adorable, but messed up from doing too much E. Even so, he made my extension bearable. We kissed on my last night there.

On your last day at Promises, everyone sits in a circle at group and describes something about you that they admire. I don't remember the first few things said about me, but midway through, the TV actor I'd taught to eat edamame took his turn and he never stopped talking. None of it had to do with me.

That was fine. I was out of there.

I went home to my cat Eme and a resolve to stay healthy and practice the tools I'd learned in rehab, sans the twelve-step meetings, which were never on my to-do list. But I started out with a fanaticism that saw me at lunch one day with my friend Gustavo and turning down the salad dressing because it was red wine vinaigrette. I explained that since my forty-five days in rehab I was off alcohol entirely.

I'd been advised against seeing or speaking to my mom until I'd reacclimated to New York, a nebulous time period they would monitor based on my behavior. But I told them what they could do with their advice. Although my dad had kept Mom informed while I was in rehab, I hadn't spoken to her for two months or more. In that time, I had done some serious navel-gazing in therapy. I'd worked up questions and insights. In other words, I had a lot of shit to say to her.

After reconnecting on the phone, I met her at her apartment.

We hugged, and she complimented me on the way I looked. We sat in the kitchen. She told me what she'd been up to, and I caught her up on some of the details about rehab—the who, where, and when. Then I started in about all the stuff that I'd learned about myself: the stories, the memories, and the insights.

I hit on everything from the neglect I felt at having to walk to school in the freezing cold to my fear that I may have been sexually abused by our old babysitter's boyfriend when left alone with him. She didn't argue, fight, or ask many questions. She didn't reach out and hug me, her only child. Nor did she accept any responsibility, which she could have done. Hey, I would have argued but ultimately understood if she had said, "Mia, I didn't learn how to be a parent from my parents and so I didn't know what the fuck I was doing. But at least I tried."

Anything. But she didn't really react. She simply said, "Oh, okay."

Maybe that was the best she had to offer. I didn't tell her anything that she didn't already know. I had no idea what I expected from the talk. Whatever it was, the result was anticlimactic. I left the apartment thinking my therapist and the others at Promises may have been right. I needed to steer clear of her for a while.

Oh, I'd also told her that I'd accepted a job modeling clothes for Lane Bryant, and because she'd modeled briefly years earlier, I'd asked her for advice. "Keep your chin up," she'd said. "Wear nude underwear. And work your eyes." Good advice for myriad situations, especially the first and the third tips, which have since gotten me through many situations both good and bad.

The opportunity to model came about independent of me. In fact, I'd never thought of modeling until a girl I knew from some showbiz thing I'd worked on years earlier, in fact right after I'd first got an agent, called me while I was in rehab. She asked if I remembered her and explained that she was working for a PR agency. She'd seen my name on a list of plus-sized models for retailer Lane Bryant's new V-Girl line for teen girls. She asked if I was interested.

Without telling her that I was in rehab, I asked how my name had been put on the list initially. She didn't know.

"I don't have any experience," I said. "I've never modeled."

"I don't think it matters," she said. "Interested?"

"No."

"Really?"

At that point, I should have told her that I was in rehab and not looking for work while I tried to get my shit together. But in fact part of getting my shit together included finding a job, something to give me a sense of self-worth and purpose.

Earlier, I'd been in therapy talking about my lack of direction, complaining about the depressing series of rejections I'd experienced as an actor going on auditions, and owning how I'd fucked up in school. My therapist had suggested applying for other jobs, but the truth was nothing appealed to me and I wasn't qualified for anything.

Yet here was this girl whom I vaguely knew handing me an opportunity. Looking back, it's almost as if fate intervened.

"It also pays $5,000," she added. "You get half up front and the other half on completion of the job."

There was more. There was a fashion show and shoot. She said legendary photographer Francesco Scavullo was doing the shoot. I knew who Scavullo was and what he meant. He'd photographed my mom when she was nineteen and a Marilyn Monroe–esque beauty heating up the Warhol scene. Through a happy accident of timing, I was nearly the same age. That was cool.

But best of all was the payday. I hadn't made a dime on my own in my life. I didn't see myself as a spoiled daddy's girl, but I was aware that I'd benefited from my dad's generosity with his gold card. Over the years, I'd used it to buy clothes, drugs, and meals at nice restaurants. It had been my safety net. But at the end of the day, I didn't have any money of my own.

From the work I was doing in rehab, I knew that, even though I thought modeling was stupid and I didn't want to do it, I'd feel better about myself for accomplishing something on my own. I told her that I was out of town, but to count me in, and that I'd call her when I got back to New York.

"It's not a done deal," she cautioned. "But it's going to help when I tell them that you're interested."

I had no idea that a new chapter of my life was about to start, but I hung up after promising to call her when I got back and felt something new, something I hadn't felt too many times before, and that was gratitude, hope, and purpose.

TWENTY-SIX

I'm Not a Model

It was August of '98, and I'd been back in New York for a few weeks when the girl from the PR agency called to inform me that I'd made the final cut as one of Lane Bryant's six V-Girls, so named after their Venezia jean line. I was thrilled. The shoot with Scavullo for the ad campaign took place soon after. I went to the studio and met the others, including top professionals like Sophie Dahl and Kate Dillon, and of course Scavullo.

Scavullo worked quickly, knowing what he wanted, and everyone was lovely, behaved, and, well, businesslike. There were lots of cell phone conversations between setups. As the only non-pro on the set, I felt intimidated and kept to myself. Things happened as I'd imagined. There was makeup and fussing by stylists. I wasn't especially comfortable being in the lights. Standing out wasn't my idea of fun. All in all, it was . . . uh, different. The whole day went by in a blur.

Almost immediately after the photo shoot, the V line debuted in a runway fashion show under a giant tent at Chelsea Piers. It was a huge, glittery event, part of the industry's annual Fashion Week. It was significant for extending the trend of marketing plus-sized fashion from women to girls. It had only been a few years since models Emme and Natalie Laughlin had helped the fashion industry discover larger women—some sixty-five million of whom were size twelve and up. The V line acknowledged the number of plus-sized girls in their teens and early twenties who didn't identify with Kate Moss or the other size-0 and -1 models on the covers of magazines.

I was floored to be part of the event, but my immediate goal was to get through it. The six of us wore jeans and a T-shirt that said V-GIRL. In addition to having fittings earlier in the week, we rehearsed the day of the show. There wasn't much to rehearse, though. We stood in the center of the stage while other models walked around us. It was nothing like the elaborate shoots I'd do later on. But I thought, *Fine, at least I don't have to worry about tripping.*

Like the photo shoot, everyone seemed to grab at me for either a touch of makeup, a brush of my hair, an assessing look, something. As I'd discover with any fashion show, there was an electric nervousness beforehand. I also did press, and I found myself surprised by the enjoyment I got from the attention—and talking!

I'd grown up seeing my dad expertly entertain reporters with his gift for coming up with the clever quip, and now I was the object of attention. I loved it. I finally had something that was my own. Reporters asked questions and took down what I said, as if it mattered. It was like a magic power—and the reason I would continue to model for Lane Bryant. I liked the way I felt.

"What are your thoughts on being a plus-sized model?" a reporter asked.

A few days earlier we'd had some media training about the V line, but none of that pertained to the questions reporters asked me. Nor had I thought about what it meant to be plus-sized rather than . . . rather than what? Skinny? Super skinny? Small? Petite? Someone who enjoyed a meal rather than constantly dieted or pushed food away? Someone who accepted the body with which she'd been born? I hadn't thought about any of these things yet. So I just said what I felt inside.

"I grew up in New Hampshire," I said, "and everybody's kind of big in New Hampshire."

There was laughter from the writers standing around me.

"But how do you feel about not looking like one of the stereotypical skinny models we see in—"

"I've always been okay with myself—physically," I said, adding the qualifier that referred to my recent stint in rehab.

Reporters also wanted to know about my dad, who was seated out in front with Teresa, Chelsea (looking gorgeous and model-like in a green print dress), and Liv (who had a cute, boyish haircut). I hadn't invited my mom. One of the writers cracked that the Tylers in the front row had bigger lips than most of the models.

"Duh," I said laughingly. "During my whole childhood, I got made fun of because of my lips. They're the family lips."

To me, the fashion show itself was much ado about nothing, as it simply required the six of us V-Girls to do little more than stand in the center of the runway while other Lane Bryant models showing additional lines did much more in terms of walking and turning. I felt stupid. To my surprise, though, we were a hit, and afterward Kate Dillon introduced me to a stylish woman named Melissa, her agent from the Wilhelmina Agency.

"We want to sign you," Melissa said.

"I'm sorry, I'm not a model," I said. "I just did this because a friend called. I don't know if I'm interested in this stuff."

"Just come in," she said, handing me her card.

I couldn't ignore her on account of inconvenience. The Wilhelmina Agency was located a half block away from my apartment. I walked in two weeks after the fashion show and met with Melissa and several other agents in the Ten-20 division for plus-sized models. Within ten minutes, they gave me a contract, reiterating their desire to sign me and describing the potential they saw for me as a model. They mentioned money and travel, working with top photographers.

"I don't know if that's what I see myself doing in the future," I said.

The agents were nice and patient. They were accustomed to dealing with all sorts of girls.

"This isn't the rest of your life," Melissa said. "It's an opportunity for right now." She smiled. "Take the contract home. Think about it."

"But I'm not signing," I said.

I was nervous about such a commitment. It seemed too adult for me.

"Just take it with you," she said. "Call me with any questions, anything you want to talk over."

I wanted to get out of their office. The light in there was extremely bright and unforgiving, white and harsh. I thought it was strange until I realized it was probably intentional, allowing the agents to see every blemish in the girls they met, and that made me more uncomfortable.

"Okay, I'll think about it," I said, taking the contract.

At home, I put the contract on my kitchen counter and tried to forget about it. I still felt too lost and directionless to make such a decision easily. I had the same fear and anxiety as a college freshman or sophomore considering a major. How do you make such a big decision when you don't know? You don't, at least I didn't, without fretting, drinking lots of coffee, and smoking lots of cigarettes.

But that contract was like a five-hundred-pound elephant in my small apartment. One night Gillian and I came in from a club and she read the contract.

"What's up with this?" she asked. "Why isn't it signed?"

"I don't want to," I said.

She gave me a look.

"Are you a fucking idiot?" she said. "Are you for real? You don't want to do this?"

I told her my reasons.

"You're an idiot, Tallarico," she said. "Wilhelmina is offering you a contract, something most people kill for. It's going to be easy money. You just made five thousand dollars doing nothing. Tell me the problem with that again."

I was unable to think of a response.

"My point exactly," she said.

TWENTY-SEVEN

Plus-sized

A few days later, I went back to the agency, holding my contract. I threw it on Melissa's desk. Grinning, I said, "Okay, I signed it." She gave me a hug. I didn't care about modeling as much as I relished the feeling of being wanted. The job started out in an unexpected way. My career took off instantly.

Seriously, I thought that I'd have to go through a process of auditions and rejections similar to the way I'd done as an actress. But no, it was different. The process was different, and the rejections I feared never materialized. In March 1998, I scored my first editorial feature in *Seventeen* magazine. I was also the first plus-sized model to appear in that magazine.

It was the magazine's prom-themed edition. I was one of seven girls flown to Los Angeles. We were put up in hotels and driven to the location at the beach. There were tents, trailers, makeup artists, stylists, a creative director, the whole army of people who're found on a shoot. I was impressed.

They had us pose on the beach in prom dresses. We wore cute dresses and laughed as we romped on the beach. To my amazement, I enjoyed myself. What was not to enjoy? We were in L.A., on the beach, the food was great, the hotel was nice, and the crew was fun. My only complaint was a super-queeny hairstylist who pulled my hair too hard and nearly yanked my head off my neck.

After someone whispered to him that I was Steven Tyler's daughter, he was a lot gentler. I don't know why that mattered to him, but it did. As for me, I learned to appreciate the stylists and makeup artists. They're the people who really make you look good in front of the camera.

I promoted that issue of *Seventeen* on *The Howie Mandel Show*. It was my first talk show appearance. Having heard Howie was a germaphobe who didn't shake hands, I'd decided it would be funny to pretend I was sick when I came on and do everything I could to shake his hand. But I nixed that after really getting sick the night before and coughing all the way to the studio. Ironically, Howie shook my hand anyway. Once off-camera, though, he pulled a bottle of Purell hand sanitizer from his desk drawer and squirted it into his palms.

Other magazine appearances followed in *Teen People*, *Us*, *Mode*, and *Moxie Girl*. I understood the attention was based on me being Steven Tyler's daughter. It was the door opener my mother had talked about years earlier. Liv had gone through the same thing. Reporters asked about my dad, and they looked disappointed when, instead of telling lurid tales of outrageous behavior around the breakfast table, of which I had none, I described him as a cute little boy in an old man's skin who I envisioned rocking out when he was eighty, with scarves tied around his walker.

But I also had a story separate from my dad, something I hadn't spent much time thinking about before. Suddenly the position I'd put myself in forced me to think about who I was, what my story was, how I felt, and what I did with my time, what I wanted to do with my life, what I believed in . . . everything. Dozens of questions were thrown at me that I'd never had to answer, let alone consider.

At nineteen, it was hard to formulate a story. I would look in the mirror or at my reflection in store windows and think, *Huh, so what's the deal?* Though I had something to do, I still felt lost and directionless. I'd started smoking pot again and drinking, but it was under control. I didn't party till obliteration. I really wanted to figure myself out. The job ended up helping.

I'd never had an issue with my body or size. Even when I went to fat camp, that was about my mom, not me. But as I was asked question after question about my size—because, after all, I was modeling a plus-sized line—it put me in a place where I was able to see something about myself that I hadn't articulated. I was different. I was an outsider. I didn't fit the ideal—whatever that was. And I was cool with that.

It was as if some protective layers had been peeled away and a picture started to emerge. At five-seven and 180 or so pounds, I had curves and heft. Some people described it as a presence; I was fine with that, too. One thing was sure: I wasn't sample size. I didn't look like a cheerleader or the hot young flavor of the month on TV. Nor did I feel like one. Nor did I care. For better or worse, I was me.

As I told people, just being me was hard enough. I was trying to figure me out. I didn't need the unrealistic burden of trying to look like someone else. Although it was strange to hear Wilhelmina tout me as a role model for girls who'd never be a size 6—I mean, just the idea of being a role model freaked me out—I was comfortable delivering the message that beauty came in all sizes, shapes, and packages. It was an important message. It was true, too.

There was something slightly rebellious about standing up for nonconformity, for being yourself, and I was a natural. It was in my genes, I suppose. But I was unprepared for how touchy the subject could be as it related to weight. I was guesting on Roseanne Barr's talk show. Growing up I'd watched Roseanne's series. I'd envied the Connor family and wished Roseanne could be my mom. So meeting her when I came on her talk show was an exciting moment.

Plus Roseanne had a serious interest in the issue I was there to discuss. She'd battled a weight problem most of her life and spoke about having undergone an operation to have a band put around her stomach so she'd eat less and lose weight. She applauded me for being the first plus-sized model in *Seventeen*. But then two women in the front row heckled me. Large-sized themselves, they didn't think being a size 12 qualified me as plus-sized.

"Hey, I'm not here trying to represent anyone but me," I said. "If you're my size, then that's who I'm representing. I'm not trying to be skinny. I'm not trying to be overweight. I'm just trying to be me."

"Yeah, well put," said Roseanne, who then pointed at the two hecklers and added, "And the two of you—shut up!"

All the Lane Bryant catalog shoots used multiple girls, typically between seven and ten, and always the same group. They needed the blonde, the brunette, the redhead, the black girl, and so on. Kate Dillon was the redhead. Philippa Allam was the blonde. Randi Graves was the black girl. And I was the brunette. I'd always heard about the catfights and jealous sniping that went on behind the scenes between models, but nothing like that happened on our sets. Ours were diva-free shoots. All of us got on well—probably because we ate the delicious catered food.

I clicked with Kate, who'd ushered me into Wilhelmina. Another girl, Jessie, was naughtier, and we found each other. It was on my first big catalog shoot, and Jessie and I were at the coffee bar. I made a comment about pot and her ears perked up. We went out back, smoked a bowl, and had a nice chat about the business, which put me at ease among these far more seasoned professionals.

Inside, I watched Jessie do her thing in front of the camera. She was posed in front of a window that was covered with a clear paper in lieu of glass so she could pop her head through it. I noticed that as she broke through the window she made a certain face, an animated look between a smile and surprise, and I thought, *Oh, that's what modeling is about. You have to do something; you need to have a look.*

So I did that same thing, and to be honest, I mimicked everything else Jessie did. Initially, I got all my moves from watching her. But the more I did, the more I developed my own thing, which was really a matter of letting my personality surface in response to a variety of situations. And there were tricks of the trade. For one photo, Kate and I were trying to listen through a wall to a conversation between Jessie and Philippa. All of us were supposed to be laughing. And the photographer said, "Sing!"

I turned to Kate.

"Sing?"

Everyone started singing. *La-la-la-la . . .*

Even though I felt stupid, I joined in.

"It makes your face animated," Kate said afterward.

At most shoots we were singing or laughing, or sometimes pretending to sing or laugh without actually making sounds. So I watched, learned, and eventually came up with my own expressions. I had my side smirk, where I smiled by raising only one cheek. That was my "Magnum." I did it on either side. That was pretty much my main move outside of showing off my boobs. It seemed that I was the first one at every shoot to ask if I could do it topless and just hold my boobs. I wasn't inhibited.

In January of '99, I walked the runway for the first time. (I didn't count my debut since it only required standing, not walking.) This—a preview of Lane Bryant's spring line for store managers in Columbus, Ohio—was a real fashion show. There was no special training. Beforehand, they simply told me to walk slow. They also had me practice in my backless heels. I wouldn't have wanted to do that on *America's Next Top Model,* but I made it without a stumble. Tyra would've approved.

Besides the attention, it didn't take me long to discover the perks of modeling, including nice hotels, travel, and free clothes. In addition to Lane Bryant's latest, my closet was full of Fubu, Vivienne Tam, and BCBG. But I was a slob, a victim of a challenging schedule. My everyday clothes were piled up on the floor opposite my bed. I lived out of my giant purse, which on any given day was crammed with the latest issue of *Rolling Stone,* the *New York Post,* my Walkman, tapes, my Wilhelmina schedule, skin cream, lip gloss, and my cell phone.

Gillian had been right about the money in modeling. It was good—and it seemed easy. With my earnings, I moved to another duplex, this one brighter and bigger, on Twelfth Avenue between Second and Third streets. Unlike my first apartment, which had basically been a safe haven from the streets, I picked this place out and decorated it myself with a couple couches, a nice TV, and a bedroom set. I was proud of it.

As good as things were, I was still reckless. One night Gillian and I smoked out on hash, and I wanted to capture what I thought was our brilliant bantering while under the influence. I set up a movie camera across from the TV and pointed it at the two couches. A couple days passed before I played back the tape, and I was thoroughly amused not by our intelligence and wit but our stupidity.

By the end of the tape, we were in our bras, laughing, complaining about the heat, and talking nonsensical shit. In the middle of a rant, Gillian heard the song "Connection 17" come on the radio and she jumped up.

"It's so trippy that song came on," she said.

"Why? It's not even a good song."

"No, it's cool because you just connected with a seventeen-year-old."

"Oh, yeah."

It was one of those you-had-to-be-there stoner references. I laughed—probably because I had been there, and I understood.

A few days earlier, I'd taken the virginity of a seventeen-year-old boy. His name was Eric, and he ran in our circle. We were at a club one night with some friends and the subject came around to sex and how each of us had lost our virginity. We went around in a circle, reliving the details. I told my story of doing it on my mother's bed with Carmen Electra playing in the background. Because I was ballsy, uninhibited, and buzzed, I added a virginity-related anecdote about how I'd once done it with a friend to ensure that his first time was great.

"He was hot and Italian," I said, laughing. "We went to his rich friend's house, smoked out of this humongous six-foot bong, went into the library, pulled out a sleeper sofa, and did it."

Then it was Eric's turn. He hesitated under the heat of our collective stares. All of us were thinking the same thing. Suddenly he looked at me.

"So what about me?" Eric said. "I'm a virgin. What about doing the same thing with me?"

Both his admission and his question took me by surprise, and it's pretty hard to shock me. Now it was my turn to be stared at. I felt the glare as I thought. Then I looked up at the gang and slowly swung around till I locked eyes with Eric. I grinned, a naughty but nice grin.

"I'll do it," I said.

He came to my place after the club. Some of the buzz from the club had worn off. So had some of my enthusiasm. In the context of the situation this may sound odd, but I'm not a slut. I've made out with plenty of guys, but I've never gone in for promiscuous, unprotected sex. At least this was one of those times when I knew I didn't have to worry about any diseases. But as I chatted with Eric, I knew I couldn't do it sober. It was too awkward. So we sent for some forties. By the time they were delivered, I'd tacked scarves over the windows to block out the sun that was starting to come up. I didn't want to see anything.

As for Eric, well, he didn't care if I was drunk, sober, in the light, or standing on my head in the closet. He was a guy about to do it for the first time.

"What are you thinking?" I asked.

"I'm nervous," he said.

"Don't be," I said, letting my fingers caress the back of his shoulders while I crossed the room to my five-disc changer. After flipping the light off, I put on DJ Shadow, hit Play, and gave him an experience that he later swore he'd remember for the rest of his life.

TWENTY-EIGHT

My Time in the Sun

Through sheer recklessness, I came close to derailing my career. It was on a winter trip to Florida for *Seventeen* magazine, and I hooked up with Gillian's friend Mike. Like me, he was almost twenty-one. He had the look and style of a Japanese gangster, but he was funny and his edginess intrigued me. After I invited him to go to Florida with me, he invited his crew, including Gillian and her sister Jocie.

Suddenly my modeling job turned into a group of eight downtown guys and girls looking to party in the sun. It wasn't a good combination from the start.

Mike and his crew arrived first. Gillian took the bus from New York City. I had first-class tickets courtesy of the shoot. Gillian, Mike, and the others were standing in front of the hotel when I pulled up in a taxi. Laughingly, we discovered that each of us had brought a bag of E. We had enough to turn on most of South Beach.

The hotel was right on the sand of South Beach. As the bellman took my bags, Gillian said, "Let's go to the beach." Before I replied, she put two hits of E in my mouth. After that, what choice did I have?

"Okay, let's go," I said.

For the next few days we got crazy. South Beach was a twenty-four-hour party, and we did our best to ensure we didn't miss any of those hours. One night, as Gillian and I walked down the street, I stopped and gave my friend a panicked look.

"I think a ghost just walked right through me," I said. "My heart is fluttering."

She cupped her face in her hands. "I didn't say anything, but last night at the club, I saw breasts—giant boobies—grow out of the DJ's record table," she said. "He was spinning boobies."

"This is bad," I said.

"We have to stop doing so much E," she said.

But we didn't take our own advice. The day before my shoot we moved into the Delano Hotel, the luxurious landmark situated right on the beach. Everyone piled into my large suite. While the guys cruised the sand, Gillian and I laid out, popped some E, and got more fucked up. Our rule was, for every two hits of E, we also took half of a quaalude. I don't know why I thought that was fun or smart. A few months earlier, that same combination had been responsible for the dragon tattoo on my back. I'd gotten it one night in New York, but I had no recollection of any of it. The only reason I knew was the shop put up a photo of me getting the work.

That day on the beach in Miami turned into a similar experience in that I suffered voids in my memory as to where the hours went. Between the sun, alcohol, E, and quaaludes, I ended up back at the hotel with severe sun poisoning. I didn't even know such a thing existed, and I wished I'd never found out.

Whatever I'd ingested was phototoxic. Aside from turning lobster red, my skin blistered, swelled, itched, and hurt. I cried just breathing in and out. The Delano was known for its luxurious all-white rooms. Lying in mine, it looked as if I'd died and gone to heaven—except it felt like hell.

I screamed in pain as I peeled off my clothes. Taking a shower was worse. Gillian wanted to help but didn't know what to do. I sent her to the store to buy whatever ointments and creams advertised themselves as relief for painful sunburn. Nothing worked. In fact, they made me feel worse. I pleaded with her to go back and find something else. At one point, I hallucinated from the pain. I looked out the hotel room window and saw Dumbo flying outside.

"Gillian," I said. "Call my dad."

"Really?" she asked.

"Tell him what's going on and that I think I'm losing my mind," I said.

Gillian used my cell phone and got ahold of my dad. From my semi-coherent state on the cool sheets of my bed, I heard her say something along the lines of "Mia's going crazy again." Then she handed the phone to me. I repeated the story with a few additional details, including the Dumbo sighting.

My dad was calm. He realized I was suffering from more than severe sunburn. He advised using Noxzema skin cream, drinking water, and resting indoors. The latter was not a problem. Gillian bought a couple jars of Noxzema and applied it all over my skin. I lay in the bed all night covered in salve like a patient in a burn ward. My shoot was the next day.

God, I freaked out all night, sleeping in fits from pain and anxiety. Before leaving my room, I looked in the mirror. It was not a good sight. Though less blistered, I was beet red. As I walked through the lobby, I looked like a lobster after an all-night costume party. At the shoot, the art director and photographer gave me long, hard, disapproving looks, but no one said anything, thank God.

I was punished enough by the shoot itself. It required me to ride a horse wearing a skirt and a denim jacket. With my sunburn and blisters, it was torture. The picture that ran months later was small and doctored to make me look less red. The talking-to I got from my agent made me feel even smaller.

In the meantime, while I'd been recovering in my room and then working, my friends ran amok at the hotel. One of Mike's friends, a hooker-like girl he'd picked up, had taken one of my extra guest cards, signed it Candy Cane, and used it to charge everything from drinks to Jet Ski rentals to lobster and steak dinners to my room. They also cleaned out the minibar and convenience baskets. They stripped the place.

A week later, after I was back home and trying to forget the debacle, the phone rang and my agent asked if I'd charged $10,000 to my room at the Delano. I hadn't bought anything other than sunburn medications. That was a huge sum of money. I took a moment to think.

"No," I said. "I maybe charged three hundred bucks' worth of stuff."

"Well, who is Candy Cane?"

Again, I paused to think.

"I don't know what you're talking about," I said.

It took some time before I figured it out. Not coincidentally *Seventeen* didn't hire me again for nearly two years—until their department underwent a change of regime and the new people wanted me. By then, I was more responsible and professional. But that trip nearly ruined my career. The funny thing was, in the back of my mind, I was thinking about getting out of the business.

Don't get me wrong. I enjoyed the attention and the perks. They knew me at Barney's and I was able to get a table at Balthazar for Sunday brunch without calling for a reservation. I was invited to hot parties, and I christened every new boutique in Soho with my credit card. I became a boldface name in the gossip columns on my own account, not because I was Steven Tyler's daughter.

That registered with me. The perks I got were based on work I did. They had nothing to do with my dad. They made me feel good about myself. I wasn't cutting, and, while I obviously got high, and sometimes too high, I stayed away from coke, which I knew wielded power over me and was a one-way ticket to tragedy.

As for my mom, I didn't share much with her. That relationship was on a low flame. But as I climbed the ranks of modeling, I still wondered what I was doing with my life. Though the money was stupid good, I didn't have the temperament for the lifestyle, for jumping on planes, checking into a hotel in a city where I didn't know anyone, eating alone, worrying about return flights, and then reconnecting with friends when I got back home.

My dissatisfaction was like a low-level hum, and yet others felt that I was on the verge of something important. One day Wilhelmina's director and co-owner, Dieter Esch, called me in for a meeting. A bankerish-looking man, his office reflected his power and importance. He told me to relax and said I was doing extremely well, that everyone was proud of me and the clients were happy. He explained that I'd reached a juncture that few models got to, and therefore it was time for me to hear what he described as his "supermodel talk."

I was flattered and embarrassed, especially given some of the thoughts I was having about modeling in general. But it was nice to be welcomed and praised, something relatively new to me. Even though I would've been last in line of those who considered me a supermodel, Dieter's opinion said otherwise. Having heard about Miami, the gist of his talk was about personal responsibility. He didn't go into detail, but I detected notes of both concern and caution in his voice.

Looking back, I get it. Dieter and the other agents were used to dealing with girls who shared a certain quality of beauty and attractiveness, a quality that bestowed itself in absolute randomness, and thus they also dealt with girls from every sort of background, including those who'd received little to no parenting, abuse, or God knows what kind of upbringing. So, in hindsight, his "supermodel" talk could also be interpreted as a veiled life lesson, more like the talk you should've received from your parents but perhaps didn't.

Dieter covered public behavior, drugs, how to deal with the press, stalkers, and even jail mail—letters written to us from prisoners, of which there was a considerable amount. As he said, I didn't have to respond. I just had to listen. Whether I remained a model or not, it was valuable stuff that I've drawn from ever since, and I appreciated that he took the time.

• • •

A short while later, actually that summer of 1999, came an unexpected diversion. I starred in *A Little Bit of Lipstick*, a low-budget independent movie about a girl from Connecticut battling insecurities about her body. In the end, she wins her guy's heart, and all it took was a little bit of lipstick. It was cute. The writer-director, J.T. Foster, had penned the script with me in mind. I got as involved as I could both in front of the camera and behind it. I helped to cast the movie. I even got Bogush a part.

Having Bogush around during the low-budget production kept the long, no-frills days and nights fun and light, and it also resulted in a joke on me. Since we met in camp, I'd always wanted to kiss him. But because we were more like brother and sister, we never did. However, one of the scenes in the movie called for us to kiss. It was a small, polite kiss on the lips, nothing passionate, so I didn't get weird or nervous. Afterward, the director asked us to do another take of the scene. I had no idea that Bogush had put him up to it. And this time, instead of a light kiss on the lips as we'd done previously, he tried to stick his tongue down my throat. It was so funny.

Following the movie, I dated the director's cousin for a while and went back to modeling. With all the running around I did, I was grateful for whoever designed purses big enough to hold what seemed like an entire closet's worth of clothes. While I was between jobs, my friend Kes contacted me. Two years younger than me, she was actually the daughter of a friend of my mom's, another child of a rocker. She'd stayed briefly with us when she was fourteen and having problems at home.

Now, at nineteen, she was grown up, and once again she needed a place to stay. Kes wouldn't have been my first choice, but taking on a roommate seemed like a good idea with all the traveling I did. It would give my place some stability, I thought. There'd be someone to talk to as I flitted in and out. Also, I wouldn't have to constantly ask friends to stop by and feed my cat. I told Kes to bring her shit over.

I overlooked the reason she hadn't continued living with my mom and me years earlier. Having raised herself, she had been like a feral cat, and after she moved in with me, I discovered she was no more tame. However, at first, she seemed like a good time. A striking girl, she was a stripper at several low-end gentlemen's clubs. That intrigued me, and I let her show me that world. It wasn't hard-core; it was stripping, and I liked the girls. They smelled good, looked pretty, and were in great shape.

I also noticed the way the girls were in total control when they gave lap dances. I was intrigued by the way they interacted with their customers, and I learned their tricks. According to Kes, the first thing the girls did when giving a lap dance was check the tags inside the guy's clothes. If it was a designer brand, they were all over them. If it was a discount chain, they went through the motions and moved on.

Kes had a large Russian clientele, and she regularly came home with fur coats, expensive shoes, and jewelry, presents from her "boyfriends." I noticed that she was often busier during the day than she was when she *worked* at night, and I asked what was up with that. Day dates, she explained, were big among strippers. She'd meet one of her nighttime admirers for lunch, typically at a restaurant she chose in a neighborhood where she had stuff on hold at stores. After lunch, they'd stroll into a store and she'd "find" a jacket or a bracelet that she loved.

"And what else is involved?" I asked.

"All men are the same," she said. "They talk through their wallet and think with their—"

"Yuck."

She shrugged at me.

"I'm not a big-time model who gets free clothes," she said.

Kes and I dressed up when we went out, and the strippers flocked to us. She knew many of them. Sometimes I bought myself lap dances. Even though I wasn't into chicks, I liked the idea of getting a lap dance from a hot woman and being sexual in a sex place.

The women knew I wasn't there to abuse or act disgusting to them. I wanted a good time. Kes and I bought bottles. The cash flowed. We had fun, and it drove the guys watching absolutely crazy.

That itself was a turn-on. If I saw a cute guy hanging out in the strip club with his buddies I would send him a girl. After his lap dance, he would run over to meet me. It was guaranteed. None of those guys recognized me. All of them wanted to know if I was a stripper. When I said no, they got even more excited.

It was a game, a cruel power trip that was emotionally safe. I made them fall in love with me and then crushed their hearts.

One night, I sent a handsome guy a lap dance. As expected, he came over after and we hung out together at the club. He made a good impression on me. Before I left, I gave him my phone number. He called an hour later. I didn't pick up, but we ended up meeting the following Saturday night, and then I brought him back to my place. We were getting romantic when he said that he had a girlfriend and couldn't do more than make out with me until he broke up with her.

"You have a girlfriend?" I asked, stunned. "If that's the case, we shouldn't even be making out."

He started to say something. I held up my hand, indicating for him to stop. I glanced at the clock.

"What time is it?" he asked.

"Time to make a decision," I said.

He took out his cell phone, went into the bathroom for privacy, and broke up with his girlfriend. Then he came out and grabbed me with a fervor that let me know that he wanted me. I got off on the power that I'd exercised over him, causing him to break up with his girlfriend just so he could be with me. In the back of my mind, though, I knew what both of us had done was fucked up.

I got my comeuppance, though. It turned out he'd lied to me, playing me as much as I'd played him. After I'd told him that I was into Spanish and Puerto Rican men, he'd given me a Latino name. It was made up. Through Kes, I found out that he was really a Turkish lowlife named Yuri. I refused to see him again. For a week, he called ten times a day, leaving the same message: why won't you talk to me?

Threats followed, and I got scared of the world Kes had ushered me into. It had started out fun and seemingly innocent, but it took me into a place where I didn't want to be. She hung out with Russian gangsters, did too many drugs, and brought girls back to my house. She didn't pay her share of the phone bill, which was exorbitant thanks to a boyfriend in Las Vegas. In other words, she was high-maintenance.

Then I had to go out of town on a modeling assignment. I laid down some simple rules for her to follow. She broke every one of them. The night before I returned, she brought a girl back to the apartment. The girl did blow in the bathroom, and when she came out Kes accused her of stealing money and they got in a physical fight. After noticing a photo of Liv and me and finding out it was my apartment, she refused to leave, causing Kes to call the cops, who found the chick in a nearby stairwell bleeding profusely from her arm, the result of a self-inflicted wound with a key.

After all that, I came home and overheard Kes in the bathroom talking shit about me to her boyfriend in Las Vegas. It was a mess. She was hanging out with a bad crowd, and by proxy so was I. I thought back to Dieter's "supermodel" talk. It made more sense than ever. She had to go.

TWENTY-NINE

Fan Mail

My success drove a wedge further between my mom and me. Still a young woman in her late forties, she had spent twenty years denying reality, fighting with my dad, and being angry at life rather than re-creating herself. Mentally and financially, it left her in a bad place—and, as would anger me most of all, wasting her life.

How many times had I yelled at her to let it go already? *Let it go!* I can still hear my voice echoing throughout the apartment after one of her rants about my dad, his money, her lack of it, and the unfairness of life. It amazed me that she still harped on the same thing nearly twenty years after they'd split. It shouldn't have been that way. After we moved to New York, she could've made something of herself.

I've gone back and looked at pictures of her at events with old pals like Warhol friend and photographer Billy Name, and they show a woman whose face retained a natural beauty that could light up a room whenever she turned on her personality. I actually think she got prettier with the character of age.

She had taste, humor, creativity, and charm. I wish she'd been able to apply them to something positive. I wish she'd been able to risk failure and disappointment to find something new instead of harping on the same old shit. I wish she'd been able to let it go. Following my eighteenth birthday, we'd drifted apart, and we kept drifting through my success as a model. Though I knew she followed my career, I didn't share it in any significant way. Oh, I gave her money—but it was just money. A thousand here, two grand there, whatever she needed. She knew I didn't care about it. As long as I had a roof over my head I was fine.

But our relationship wasn't. One day in early 2000, I left her apartment feeling numb and knowing something had to change. I'd stopped by to check in on her. She'd had on the Hermès scarf that I'd given her the previous Christmas, my traditional gift to her. I'd told her that she looked good. While talking, I'd caught her up on how I'd spent my birthday and the holidays at my dad's, which had led to some intense questioning and then into a diatribe about all that my dad had and how little she had, how unfair it all was and, as I'd told her, the same old yadda-yadda-yadda.

After all these years, I liked to think that I'd learned how to speak to her calmly and unemotionally. We'd reached a détente in our everyday lives. Except when—or until—my dad was injected into the conversation. Then both of us lost control, first she and then I. And that's what happened again. All hell broke loose, and the fight turned out to be my breaking point.

"I can't take it anymore," I said.

"You?" she said. "Did you hear what I said? It doesn't have anything to do with you. It's about me and not getting what I deserved."

As I said, yadda-yadda-yadda. My mom's suffering made me feel terrible. Her pain was contagious. It was as if she injected it straight into my veins. As I left the apartment that afternoon, something clicked inside me and I knew that for the sake of my own sanity I had to cut myself off from her, and I did.

Modeling was also a source of confusion and aggravation. I sound spoiled and ungrateful to utter a single syllable of complaint against a job that, after three years of nearly nonstop work, had begun to pay me $20,000 to $30,000 a shoot. The plus-sized world had taken off, and I was a beneficiary. I'd been featured in *Jane*, *Glamour*, *Teen*, and *Jump*, but the job didn't seem to fit.

I was becoming temperamental, and that wasn't me. I nearly walked out of one shoot where I had to pretend there was a bird in my hand. They planned on Photoshopping it in later. The photographer asked if I could act like a bird.

"Act like a bird?" I said.

"Yes," he replied. "Light. Feathery. Tweet-tweet."

I stood perfectly still as I considered his request.

"What kind of bird?" I asked.

"Light and feathery," he repeated.

I didn't know whether to laugh or to say something like, "How about I turn into a big angry bird that flies the fuck out of here?" I didn't do either. I took a break, smoked a cig, and then pretended I was a bird.

I didn't understand my disenchantment with the work, why I wasn't connecting with it. I tried injecting more of myself in shoots, more of my personality. I even started to bring my own makeup and accessories. To my surprise, my suggestions were usually appreciated. The art directors and photographers liked my fire. Lane Bryant even created a rocker-themed campaign for me with jeans and black tank tops. In the photo shoot, I led a gang of girls. It was closer to me.

But I still didn't feel connected to the work. Part of modeling is allowing yourself to be disconnected from your real self so that the photographer can use you in whatever way fits the shoot, the clothes, and the client's vision. After all, you are modeling. That's why you can't take the job too seriously or too personally, and believe me, some of the people I met at those shoots were among the most critical and caustic individuals I've ever met.

One time someone pointed at me and said, "Oh fuck, look at the fucking tattoo on her back. Why didn't someone tell me about the fucking tattoo?" I felt my temper surge, and my inclination was to say, "Excuse me, but that's *my* fucking back you're talking about, and it's a part of *me*!" But I kept quiet. You have to let it go. As they said in *The Godfather*, it's not personal. It's business.

On the other hand, that's what bugged me about modeling. It wasn't personal, and what I didn't understand until later was that I needed to feel it was personal in order to make it seem as if it mattered.

Then I did a photo shoot and interview for *USA Weekend*. The photo shoot was a disaster. I'd been told to bring my own clothes, but the photographer didn't like what I brought. Then I had a disagreement with the makeup artist over how she wanted to do my face. Then the photographer suggested one unflattering pose after another. By the end, I was fed up, maybe at the end of my career.

> That sense of mattering, that sense of purpose and significance all of us want, was missing from my life, as it had been my whole life. If something didn't matter, why the hell do it?

As I was gathering my things, the writer approached and asked if they could add a line at the end of the story telling readers that I would answer questions they had for me. The writer explained it was a last-minute idea her editor had had, based on my reputation as a role model for what she described as "normal-sized" girls. Normally I would've said sure, anything, but I was in such a bad mood that I agreed to answer just one.

"You'll have to contact me," I said.

"We will," the writer chirped.

Then I forgot about it until the story appeared and I got a call from my agent. She said the response to my offer had been overwhelming. The paper estimated it had received more than twenty thousand e-mails and letters. I was blown away. I had no idea of the nerve that I'd touched in the public or of the nerve that response would touch in me. Half of the e-mails and letters that came in were of the "I hate you" variety from women who didn't believe that as a size 10 or 12 I should pass myself off as plus-sized. The other letters praised, supported, and thanked me for being a role model.

One teenage girl wrote that she'd always been self-conscious about her body and tried to cover up by wearing layers of clothes, but after seeing me in the Lane Bryant catalog in jeans and a tank top, she put on the exact same outfit. It was the first time she'd ever worn a tank top as a teen. She wrote that I'd made her feel that she could be large *and* beautiful. "For the first time, I'm comfortable in my own skin," she added. "Thank you, Mia. Thank you so much."

Then there was the thirteen-year-old girl who'd spent the past year battling cancer. She wrote me an amazing seven-page letter. But instead of writing about her own life-threatening illness, she addressed my issues, the stuff I was struggling with. I don't have any idea how she'd picked up on them, but in her letter she told me that I should feel better about myself, not get so down, and know that I was making a difference. She then described how she got through her more difficult moments and suggested ways I could do the same thing.

> *There are beautiful things all around us every day. It may not seem like it, but they're there if you look. For me, it's a hug from my mom and dad. It can also be a pretty flower or a special song. You know what I do? I share those things with the people that I love. Like I hug my mom and dad back. Or I give them the pretty flower. That always makes me feel better.*

I was touched beyond anything that had happened to me before. Until then, I hadn't considered that my work and the related interviews might be affecting people. I knew people were looking at me, but I had no idea they were listening, too. I continued to speak out. In interviews, I said the things that I felt, not things I'd been coached to say. I told a story of how someone once asked me what clothes would help cover their stomach and make their little muffin-top disappear. "Sometimes it's better to show off that bulge instead of trying to hide it," I said. Then I'd lifted up my shirt. "I like my stomach, and I think it's sexy to have a little belly."

Asked my fashion dos and don'ts, I replied that I didn't have any specific dos, and as for don'ts, I had one that applied to everybody. "You can't be weak. That's the one thing. You have to be strong." These things were easy to come up with because I spoke from my heart. Like when I was asked what my favorite piece of clothing or accessory was. That was an easy one. "Self-esteem," I said. "It's the one thing you can't ever leave at home." I found that I liked putting myself out there.

Later I realized something about the problem I had with modeling. While I was good at saying these things, inside I often felt like a hypocrite because I knew that I wasn't as together as I sounded. With my picture in magazines and catalogs, it may have appeared that I'd arrived, but I was still a work in progress, still creating myself, still trying to find myself. But thank goodness for the opportunities I was getting.

Despite my love-hate relationship with the business, it was through modeling that I was beginning to acquire a lesson that when I look back probably saved my life, and certainly would end up directing my life. People reached out to me through e-mail and letters because they wanted to make a connection with someone they admired, someone who'd spoken to them. Unlike the groupies in my dad's world, these were positive efforts. They were substantive in terms of quality of life, why we're here, and other big questions. They mattered. They gave meaning to their lives.

I needed to do the same thing. I needed those same types of connections. I needed to find a way to reach out, too, and feel like I mattered.

MySpace

Per my morning routine, after waking up, I went straight to my desk and turned on the computer. While it booted up, I opened the small stained-glass window on the wall, letting in the day's fresh air. My first and only stop was my MySpace page, which would occupy me without a break until lunchtime. I checked my fan page, accepted new friends, set my comments, and went through the messages. There were nearly two hundred of them, and the day was just starting.

I suppose it was within minutes—though who knows since time melts and I seem to enter a world of my own when I work on the computer—but soon I had music going, questions on the screen to answer, and I was typing a message to my boyfriend Brian about some songs we'd been writing. I also made a tattoo appointment with Kari (you have to make them months in advance), and I sent the date to Brian, who'd said he wanted to come with me.

Then I began answering some of the questions people had sent. One was about a mall in Massachusetts. Another was from a girl wanting advice on getting into modeling (from the photo she sent, I saw she was pretty enough, though I laughed at the reaction I imagined from whatever agency she went to when they saw the numerous piercings on her nose, lips, and eyes). Someone else wanted the name of a song I'd played on the site a few weeks earlier, another girl wanted to know where she could find a picture of the fairy tattooed on my arm, and then there were e-mails about the tougher subjects that my site was really about, what to do when people are dealing with tough times from drugs, alcohol, weight, or abuse, or they're ready to face issues from the past.

I was in awe of MySpace. On one level, it did something so simple by giving people all the tools they need to create, host, and manage their own website. All you had to do was join the community. It was like showing up at a Grateful Dead concert with your tape recorder and being told that you were free to tape the show if you wanted. On another level, though, they made something frightening and complex easy by giving people a place of their own, a place they could call "my space," where they could go and connect with other people.

It's a parallel world, a haven that's not perfectly safe but much safer in terms of talking with other people, making and collecting friends, sharing information and interests, asking questions, and dealing with possible rejection. For me, it was more than perfect. It was essential, what I lacked and needed—and now of course maintaining this special community occupies practically all my time.

In the beginning I had my own eponymous dot-com, but nothing really happened with it until I transferred all the content to MySpace in June of '04. First I created lists of my favorite music, movies, books, and TV shows, and posted jokes. Less than three years later, some thirty thousand people had signed on as a friend and we regularly exchanged thoughts, experiences, and advice on topics from abuse and addiction to books, bad relationships, and flattering jeans. We were also there for each other. I was there for them, and they were there for me.

Initially I started the website because I felt alone, isolated, and in need of someone with whom I could talk. I had no expectations. My mom was dead, my marriage was unraveling, and I felt like an ant in the desert. I taught myself basic HTML and put up songs, pictures, and jokes that seemed pertinent. People responded to the first couple of jokes I posted. In those jokes were pearls. "Not everyone who shits on you is your enemy. Not everyone who gets you out of shit is your friend."

I didn't realize it then, but about a year into the blog, it became an expression of my life, exactly the reason I'd started it. In May of '05, I titled a blog "I Miss NYC." (I did.) The entry was a humorous list that completed the phrase "You know you're from New York City when . . ."

- *You can get into a four-hour argument on how to get from Columbus Circle to Battery Park at 3:30 on a Friday before a long weekend, but you can't find Wisconsin on a map.*

- *You say "the city" and expect everyone to know you mean Manhattan.*

- *You've gotten jaywalking down to an art form.*

- *You take a taxi to get to your health club to exercise.*

- *Your idea of personal space is no one actually standing on your toes.*

- *$50 worth of groceries fits in one paper bag.*

- *You have a minimum of five "worst cab ride ever" stories.*

- *You don't notice sirens anymore.*

- *Your doorman is Russian, your grocer is Korean, your deli man is Israeli, your building super is Italian, your laundry guy is Chinese, your favorite bartender is Irish, your favorite diner owner is Greek, the watch seller on your corner is Senegalese, your last cabbie was Pakistani, your newsstand guy is Indian, and your favorite falafel guy is Egyptian.*

In June of '05, I was getting divorced, and I posted "Some Things Every Woman Should Know." The last line had rung especially true. "They say it takes a minute to find a special person, an hour to appreciate them, a day to love them, and an entire lifetime to forget them." As I continued to post, something happened to the site. People responded. And I replied back to them. It became our special place where I found that talking to other people about their rough times was a way to help myself through my tough times. We ragged on American Idol, got someone help for alcoholism, shared videos, revealed our secrets and fears, and asked each other questions. Truths emerged. No one goes through life problem-free. No one can solve their problems by themselves.

• • •

*After lunch, I saw that there were 112 responses to my most recent post,
"Let It Go." The first one I opened underscored the importance of the
site.*

> Hi Mia,
> You don't know me. I'm Stefanie. I've been a fan of yours
> since I was 18 years old. Today you posted a small forward
> called "Let Go." I hadn't got out of bed for 3 days now and
> I'm running on saltine crackers and water. No, not because
> I'm sick but because I'm depressed. See, I've been called "fat"
> my whole life. I have been dumped because I wasn't as thin as
> a Barbie. To be honest, I never wanted to be thin. That was
> up until recently. See, he (referring to the man I've been
> seeing) told me that he wants a skinny chick to have sex with
> me. He told me as if it didn't hurt me. I've been so jaded since
> then. I've constantly looked in the mirror staring at myself
> completely naked and would sit and cry. "If only I was
> skinnier he would love me" . . . It wasn't until Saturday he
> told me I was not good enough for him (he didn't say it straight
> out, but the point was I wasn't good enough for him anymore).
>
> So I read your forward today. Today I was giving up . . . I
> thought I had lost this battle and thought life would be better
> without me. Silly of me, I know. But I read it . . . "Let Go."
> I kept reading over and over . . . Instead of giving up . . . I'm
> letting go.
>
> Mia, I want you to know you saved me today. Thank you.

There's a power that comes from putting out healing effort. When I
read that e-mail I felt stronger, more courageous, and better about myself.

Part Four

You have been criticizing yourself for years

and it hasn't worked. Try approving

of yourself and see what happens.

—*Louis L. Hay*

THIRTY

A New Boyfriend

It was fall 2000, and I was on a flight back to the United States from a modeling job in Europe, looking through a fashion magazine, when I thought about her. It had to have been the picture that inspired me; it was an ad featuring actress Catherine Deneuve. Although slightly older, she was blonde and pretty. I noticed the way her hair was pulled back, and all of a sudden I wondered what, and how, my mom was doing.

It had been almost eight months since I'd left the apartment following our blowup. In that time, I'd worked my ass off. I'd crisscrossed the Atlantic a half dozen times, going to London, Paris, and Milan. That didn't count jobs I did domestically. I'd spent too many days working and too many nights by myself, one city starting to feel like another, in that even if I cooked up an adventure it was lonely.

It was interesting how much time had passed without my thinking about her and then how in an instant I had a thousand questions—and no answers. More than interesting, it was also weird; I'd never felt like I *wanted* to see my mom.

After a day back in the city, I went to her building on Sixty-eighth Street. It was afternoon, and I showed up unannounced

after doing errands and working my way uptown. I'd taken the 6
subway, walked a couple blocks after getting off, and found myself
giving the doorman a warm hello. He asked where I'd been.

"Working," I said. "Is my mom home?"

"Yes, I think she's there," he said. "I didn't see her go out
today."

I was calm as I stepped into the elevator. Outside the door, I
took a deep breath to clear my head and told myself that seeing
her again wasn't big deal. Since I'd basically written her off, it
wasn't. She was my insane mom. She was going to be the same as
she always was. Little did I know that when the door opened I
would get one of the surprises of my life.

So I knocked on the door and when she didn't answer right
away I rang the doorbell. "Coming," she yelled from deep within
the apartment, and then I heard her footsteps across the wood
floor. A moment later, she was standing across from me, and my
mouth fell open. It didn't just fall. It was like a plummeting elevator.

"Oh my God," I said. "What happened to you?"

Grinning, my mom reached out and we hugged. She had lost
weight, and in black pants, a black cashmere sweater, and with
her hair done, she looked even better. Catherine Deneuve had
nothing on my mom. I didn't put it this way, but she looked hot. I
took a step back to give her a more careful and thorough looking-
over, almost like a reality check.

"I know," she said.

We caught up in the kitchen, talking like two friends. I kept
waiting for her to go negative on me, but she didn't. After I'd told
her about some of my travels and some stories about having taken
in Kes and then kicking her out, my mom told me to follow her
into the bedroom. She had me sit on her bed while getting something she'd forgotten in the other room. She said she was trying to
work on another book. I felt a clutch in my stomach. But it passed
when she explained this one was about her Warhol days. Then
she came back into the room and sat down next to me holding a
photo album.

"I have a new boyfriend," she said.

"I didn't know you had an old boyfriend," I said, smiling.

"You know what I mean," she said. "Do you want to see pictures of him?"

You bet I wanted to see pictures. But I didn't have to answer her question. She opened the album and started the narrative. His name was Keith Waa. In the opening photos, I saw that he was thin and lanky, had long brown hair, and had tattoos covering his arms and torso. My mom pointed out that he'd done the tattoos himself. I was speechless. He sure didn't look like one of the Upper East Side sugar daddies my mom had always mused about as the solution to her woes.

"Cool chain," I said, pointing to a heavy chain around his neck.

"He's earthy," my mom said. "What do you think?"

I didn't know what to say. My mom, who had complained all my life, had a boyfriend. She looked great. She sounded happy. She had a life. She said she was in love. *In love*. What did I think? It was like I walked into this bizzaro alternative world starring my mom.

While I was thinking of what to say, she turned the page in the photo album and looked at me.

"Ew, mom, he's naked in these pictures," I exclaimed.

"He's cute, isn't he?" she said.

"I don't know that I want to see this much," I said.

She answered all my questions. Keith was a musician. He had released an album a couple years earlier. He was also a sculptor, she said. They had met through friends. At thirty-four years old—fourteen years younger than her, she admitted proudly—he had two young children and was in the process of getting a divorce.

"Where does he live?" I asked.

"He doesn't really have a house," my mom said. "He lives in a room in a house on Staten Island."

"I guess he doesn't have a lot of stuff."

"He carries a backpack," she said. "His whole life is in that backpack. It's kind of cool, in a way."

That worried me. My mom had been out of circulation for a decade. I didn't know if she was naïve, desperate, both, or simply out of her mind. Maybe she'd fallen prey to a professional gold digger who had mistakenly thought there was gold to dig for. I got protective and reminded her of the time a year or so earlier when we'd been out and a woman had spit on her for wearing a fur coat. I'd turned around and tripped the lady and probably would've decked her if my mom hadn't pulled me away.

"Don't worry," she said, explaining that Keith treated her well and made her feel good. "Nothing wrong with that."

"Agreed," I said. "But do I have to keep looking at him naked? I haven't even met him and there's his thingie.

"Finally you do what I've been telling you to do since I was a little kid," I continued.

"What?" she asked.

"Get with a normal guy. He's exactly the kind of guy I always thought you should be with."

"I know," she said, brightening as she pointed out favorite photos and then, like a naughty girlfriend, turned over one of the naked photos again.

"Why didn't you do this twenty years ago?" I asked.

"I don't know," she said.

I knew why it had finally happened. It happened because she had stopped trying to be someone she wasn't. She had stopped trying to be Cyrinda Foxe and had gone back to being Kathleen Hetzekian. She may not have been that familiar with Kathleen after years of denying her existence, but it was a lot easier to quit pretending and be real. That was obvious. She was happy, and she looked really good.

She didn't say anything that day about having serious money troubles, but a few months later she lost her apartment. While re-grouping, she spent several days with me on Twelfth Street. Although angry and bitter, she was more accepting than I would've expected, all of which I attributed to her relationship with Keith. She sent her stuff in boxes to a friend's house in upstate New York. Sitting at my kitchen table, she joked that she'd turned into a downtown chick again.

But it was temporary. She was going to move in with Keith, into his cramped little room. I marveled at her. Here she was, a woman whose life had been spent in pursuit of status symbols, and she'd recently sold her Dior and Hermès, including scarves I'd bought her over the years, in preparation to move in with a guy whose belongings fit into a backpack.

"Mom? What's happening to you?"

"What are you going to do?" she said.

I'll always remember that night. We talked into the wee hours, and something remarkable happened. As the hours melted, my mom opened up about her relationship, her body, Keith, and their most intimate moments together. It was amazing to see her blossom in front of me, like a flower with beautiful, fragile petals, and similarly she regarded and respected me as a woman, too, which was apparent when she asked me for advice after revealing that she was hesitant when she and Keith were in bed.

"Why do you hold back?" I asked.

"Because it hurts," she said.

"Then you aren't doing it right," I said.

"Maybe I forgot how to do it," she mused.

"No," I said, laughing. "That's impossible. Everybody knows how, and no one ever forgets."

What followed was a frank and instructive talk about sex. Except that I was the teacher and she was the student. She asked how certain things were done and listened, sometimes with her eyes wide or her hand covering her embarrassed grin, as I responded in graphic detail, told her about positions, and even suggested a few things she might want to try.

By three or four a.m., my voice was gone and my mom was falling asleep on the sofa. It was the best conversation we'd ever had. It was also the most meaningful. Both of us felt good about it.

We didn't kiss, hug, and become best buddies. That would've been false. It wouldn't have been us. But for however many hours had passed, we'd pushed the bullshit to the side, talked about something important, and accomplished more in one night than we had in years.

Let It Go!

There are people who can walk away from you
and hear me when I tell you this
when people can walk away from you
Let them walk.

I don't want you to try to talk another person into
Staying with you, loving you, calling you, caring
about you, coming to see you, staying attached to you.
I mean hang up the phone.

When people can walk away from you, let them walk.
Your destiny is never tied to anybody that left.

People leave you because they are not jointed to you.
And if they are not jointed to you, you can't make them
stay. Let them go.

And it doesn't mean that they are a bad person, it
just means that their part in the story is over. And
you've got to know when people's part in your story is
over so that you don't keep trying to raise the dead.

You've got to know when it's dead. You've got to know
when it's over. Let me tell you something:

If you are holding on to something that doesn't belong
to you and was never intended for your life, then you
need to . . . LET IT GO!

If you are holding on to past hurts and pains . . .
LET IT GO!

*If someone can't treat you right, love you back, and
see your worth . . . LET IT GO!*

If someone has angered you . . . LET IT GO!

*If you are holding on to some thoughts of evil and revenge . . .
LET IT GO!*

*If you are involved in a wrong relationship or addiction . . .
LET IT GO!*

*If you are holding on to a job that no longer meets
your needs or talents . . . LET IT GO!*

If you have a bad attitude . . . LET IT GO!

*If you keep judging others to make yourself feel
better . . . LET IT GO!*

If you're stuck in the past . . . LET IT GO!

*If you're struggling with the healing of a broken
relationship . . . LET IT GO!*

*If you keep trying to help someone who won't even
try to help themselves . . . LET IT GO!*

If you're feeling depressed and stressed . . . LET IT GO!

*Let the past be the past.
Forget the former things.*

I met Keith the following weekend. The three of us went to dinner, and I stared at him the entire time, sizing him up. Between his background, which included a stint in prison; his tattoos (a thick tree with wide branches spread across his chest); his chain-link necklace; and his long hair, he was an imposing figure. I saw why my mom said normally people were scared of him. But that night he was scared of me.

He needn't have been. I saw him as my mom's guardian angel. I still had no clear idea where or how he came into her life, but I got a good feeling from him and an even better one when I heard her voice after she began staying with him in Staten Island. I know she would've preferred a Park Avenue address or even her old address on Sixty-eighth Street to living in a single room, but she remained calm and her voice even contained a gaiety that told me she was making the best of it.

She reprioritized, putting her relationship before all the other crap that used to be important to her. It was a lesson. All the things she'd held dear in the past never made her feel as good as she did when she hooked up with Keith, a guy who carried his worldly possessions in his backpack.

THIRTY-ONE

Cancer

During the eight months I didn't speak with my mom, she had been diagnosed and treated for benign tumors in her uterus. She told me about it before she moved in with Keith, adding that soon after the original diagnosis the tumors had hemorrhaged and her doctor had put her on Depo-Provera, a progestin contraceptive that decreases the output of hormones that stimulate the ovaries.

"And?" I asked, concerned.

She shrugged. As it turned out, she continued to hemorrhage. After another exam and more tests, her doctor said she needed a hysterectomy. I remember the anger in her voice when she called after she'd spoken to her doctor. Even though she was almost fifty years old and didn't plan on getting pregnant, she still freaked out and cried about losing that vital part of her womanhood. In retrospect, I think she also cried because she had an intuitive feeling the bad news would get worse.

Keith was a calming influence. I can't imagine her, or any of us, going through that situation without him, or the situation that came next. One day in March of '01, she lost control of her bladder. She was with Keith in Staten Island when that happened. As she later recalled, at first she didn't even realize that she'd peed. Then once she noticed, she was confused, as if the world had reversed its rotation and with an incredible whoosh reality had blown past her. Then nothing.

In that life-changing instant, she suffered a stroke. She didn't remember anything because there was a gap in her memory between when she peed and when her life turned into a puddle, where time literally stopped and started. I got on the computer and found out there are a number of warning signs of a stroke, including weakness or numbness in the face, arm, leg, or one side of the body; trouble walking, dizziness, loss of balance or coordination; trouble seeing with one or both eyes; confusion; trouble swallowing; and loss of bowel or bladder control.

My mom was rushed to Staten Island University Hospital. Keith called me a short time later, and I jumped in a cab. Staten Island wasn't an easy place to get to. It took me two hours to get to the hospital. On the way, I called my dad, who said to let him know any information I found out and if she needed anything.

As I passed through the hospital's front door, I had the sense of entering another phase of life. The institutional antiseptic smelled like sickness, and for some reason I knew this wasn't going to be good. I'd spent so much of my life running away, either literally or with drugs. This time there was no running away, and I got scared.

When I got to my mom's room, I found her in bed and pretty heavily sedated. Keith got up as soon as I came in and gave me a hug. I kissed my mom and asked how she was doing. It's such a stupid question to ask someone lying in bed in a hospital. If they were doing okay, they wouldn't be there. I made some crack to that end, which got a nod and a smile from my mom.

Keith then relayed as much information as the doctors had given him, and I spent time with both of them in her room until my mom dozed off. I'd like to say that I was a paragon of strength, but I wasn't. I left the hospital feeling frightened, mad, and just fucking unsure what to do. On the cab ride home, I thought, *Thank God for Keith*. Then back at my place I got obliterated on cheap wine and went for a walk.

Days later I realized how traumatized I was by my mom's stroke when I tried to recall what I'd done that night and couldn't remember much of anything. I remembered pouring Franzia wine into an empty Snapple bottle and leaving the house. But I don't know where I walked or for how long. The next thing I recalled was sitting outside my old boyfriend Sean's apartment on Twenty-third and Ninth. When I didn't find him home, I waited on the stoop outside, hoping he'd come back and take care of me.

I don't know how long I waited there or how late it got, though I remember feeling the chill of the night, but when Sean didn't materialize I called Louis, another ex-boyfriend/friend I'd dated briefly. Given that I was drunk, I don't know whether he was the first person I tried or the first person who picked up their phone that night, but God bless him, he dropped whatever he was doing, took a cab from his place in Queens, found me on the street, and took me home.

My mom, weak and scared, left the hospital after staying nearly seven days. She returned to Keith's where she convalesced without regaining her strength. At her best that spring, she needed a cane to help her walk. In April, she underwent a battery of tests at Beth Israel Hospital in the city and afterward learned the reason she wasn't getting better was that she had cancer—or more specifically, glioblastoma, the most common and aggressive type of brain tumor.

It was terrible news. Treatment options included radiation, chemotherapy, and an operation to remove the tumor. She was told that five-year survival rates were a depressingly low 3 percent. I sat on her bed in the hospital. Her voice alternated between tears, anger, and fear. It just wasn't fucking fair, she said, after telling me that her doctor had explained that glioblastomas don't usually produce symptoms, like her stroke, until they have grown large, and by then it's too late.

"What do the doctors say your chances are?" I asked.

"Eighteen months," she said.

Upon hearing that, I had no idea what to say. I stood up and walked across the room. Pictures of her CAT scans were on the table. I looked at them. They showed my mom's brain and the tumor. I turned back to her.

"That's less than two years," I said.

"It's just their guess," she said. "Treatment could work. They could be wrong."

Between modeling gigs, I spent some time videotaping bands for Sony Records. It was a creative outlet and a convenient way to meet boys. In the back of my head, I was searching for something to do after or in addition to modeling. I knew standing in front of the camera wasn't going to be a long-term pursuit of mine. But I was troubled by not knowing what else I wanted to do.

More than that troubled me, though. My mom's terminal condition had sent me into a tailspin. Although I spoke about it with Gillian, Sean, and other friends, I didn't know how to express my emotions. I had spent most of my nearly twenty-three years avoiding such feelings, deflecting or dodging them with booze, Ecstasy, pot, coke. Talking with friends, I didn't know how to get past "my mom has brain cancer and the doctor gave her eighteen months to live. We're already one month through that."

The conversations my mom and I had were stilted and difficult. I wish they hadn't been like that. But I didn't have the skills to reach out to her. The shit from the past blocked any meaningful exchanges beyond "How are you today?" and "Do you need anything?" After visiting with her, I would feel terrible. God, how pathetic is it when simply saying "I love you" isn't simple?

I was angry—angry at my mom, angry at myself, angry at the world—and I did what I'd always done when I was slammed with such feelings. I ran away. This time I left town and went to L.A., where a friend from modeling had given me a open invite to her house in the Hollywood Hills.

I wanted to take a friend. The only person available was Kes, the one person with whom I probably shouldn't have gone. That was true for a couple of reasons. First, we hadn't finished hashing out the reasons I'd kicked her out of my apartment. Then, in terms of serving as a sounding board for the issues I had with my mom, she had an even worse relationship with her mother, another faded siren from the '70s.

After cocktailing it up on the flight, we arrived at my friend's home in the hills, a modern, multilevel, multimillion-dollar palace of concrete and glass whose clean lines, sparse decor, and expansive views looked straight out of a design magazine, and yet it was so cold and isolating it felt like a freezer. Kes and I spent the week floating between trendy stores, meals, and parties. Days and nights blurred. Some of the people we hung with were familiar, but I didn't *know* anyone—and in retrospect what I needed more than anything was a comforting hug and a good cry.

One night there was a party at the house where we were staying. I went from room to room, visiting and making conversation, until I felt a switch flip inside me. It was as if reality smacked me upside the head. What was I doing at this party across the country from where I lived? I had no idea who most of the people were. All of a sudden I felt disconnected, claustrophobic, and struggling for breath.

I went outside on the balcony. Things were worse out there. The balcony was suspended over a dark ravine and the view mesmerized me as I puffed on a joint and stared into the blackness below. Soon I felt myself overwhelmed by sadness, anger, and aloneness as I dared to let myself contemplate the pain and loss of my mother. I pictured my life as one of those party balloons that's let loose and floats through the sky until it disappears into the distance. I felt like I was at that point where it's a vague dot at the end of the sky, almost out of sight.

My pity party soon turned into a contemplation of suicide as a solution to these problems. I'd jump off the balcony and put an end to my misery, I thought. No more emptiness, fear, sadness, indecision, confusion, anger, and pain. I smiled forlornly, thinking that no one would find me in the deep ravine down below. It would be days if not weeks before someone wondered where I was, and then wouldn't they be surprised? Wouldn't they miss me? Wouldn't they all be sorry?

The truly sad part was that I really wanted the opposite of everything that I was telling myself. I wanted to tell my mom that I was scared for her and hated with every fiber of my being the death sentence that she'd been given. I wanted to hug her. I also wanted to shake her and tell her that I was angry for all the years she'd wasted complaining instead of living. And when you put her complaints into the context of what she was battling, which was worse, a junky car or brain cancer? I wanted to be able to simply tell her not to die. I didn't want to be alone. I already felt too alone—and scared, confused, sad, empty . . .

It was later that I realized beyond all that I didn't want to be my mom, in the sense that I wanted my life to matter. Ultimately, that was why, after sitting on that balcony for some indeterminate length of time, I'd looked up and asked God for a sign that I should continue to live. And that's what had allowed me to appreciate the irony and relief I felt moments later when my cell phone rang with a message from an MTV executive, offering me a job as a VJ on MTV2.

After retrieving the message, I stared up at the sky full of stars and had a good laugh at the twistedness of life. In the confusion of my mom's diagnosis, I'd forgotten that I'd auditioned for the network. The timing of the news that I'd gotten the job was too weird. I told Kes and said she was welcome to stay longer, but I had to get back to New York right away. She decided to leave, too.

We caught a flight the next day and slept the entire way to New York. I woke up to the pilot's announcement that we were beginning our approach. A few minutes later, the tall buildings of the city came into view outside the window. Just as I had on the balcony the previous night, I had the sense of looking down on my life—except this time, rather than my exit, I pondered my return, and to be perfectly forthright, it scared the crap out of me.

• • •

The MTV job was relatively easy for an on-air position. They handed me a rundown of the videos scheduled to air and I'd research the bands and write my own copy. I brought my own clothes, too. As they'd promised, it really was all about me being myself. I imagine that's also why I never connected with the work, which was the number one requirement. Whenever you're in front of a camera, you have to sell it and make people feel that you believe what you're doing, and I wasn't able to sell myself. I didn't believe in what I had to sell.

Not that it mattered. By the end of the summer, MTV reconceived that block of programming without VJs. In the meantime, my mom underwent brain surgery. She'd been getting weaker. Doctors explained that removing the tumor might prolong her life, might slow or alleviate some of the rapid debilitation that was happening in front of our eyes, but ultimately the operation wouldn't save her life. Even if they removed the entire tumor, it was all but guaranteed to grow back.

"Why not?" she said when I asked if the risk was worth it. "What the fuck choice do I have?"

Her decision showed me how powerful our will to live is despite any circumstance, even one as negative as terminal brain cancer. Realizing it helped me see one of the more indelible ways all of us are connected. But we don't lose our uniqueness either, and my mom was evidence of that. She was taken into surgery early in the morning. Having spoken to her the night before, I showed up shortly before noon and waited for her to be brought out of recovery.

My friend John Bogush was with me. As we waited, a camera crew from one of the nightly entertainment TV shows joined us, and I found out that my mom had arranged for them to cover her post-op recovery. Only my insane mom! Who else would dare turn such a sad, dire moment into a photo op? I buried my head in Bogush's shoulder. I was horrified. But the cameras rolled as she was wheeled on a gurney from the elevator. Though heavily bandaged and barely conscious, she still managed a weak smile and a few words into the reporter's microphone.

The reporter then turned and insisted on interviewing me, too. In shock, or rather a state of disbelief, I gave a comment, something short and terse, and then I shooed the cameras away. I wanted my mom to get to her room!

Once again Keith was her rock. Thank God he was there. I grabbed Bogush, who kept me afloat, and told him that I had to get out of there.

"Let's go to your place," he said.

"No, I mean, I've got to get out of the country," I said.

He indulged me. I didn't want to see or smell her illness. I knew it was only going to get worse. We left the next day for Aruba. We spent nine days there, getting silly and sunburned, and then he brought me home to deal. It was time for me to grow up.

THIRTY-TWO

Amends

When I returned, I found my mom ready to leave the hospital. Since Keith lived too far from Beth Israel and she was too weak and fragile to climb up into his high platform bed, my mom moved into my place. We talked and she received lots of phone calls. It was difficult for us to share such a small space, and her illness added complications to the situation. Even though she was able to get around, it was clear that her health was going downhill.

I remember a lot of tension beneath the surface, as if the stuff we were doing grated against all that went unspoken. One day we were out and it started to rain. Cabs were impossible to find. She began to bitch and complain, and I lost my temper. I told her to shut up.

"I'm sick, you know," she snapped.

Oh God, I thought, *she's right. What am I doing?* My dad asked a similar question one day when we were talking on the phone. Hearing the anger and bitterness in my voice, he asked what I was doing about my apparent inability to deal with the stresses and emotions. Good question. I realized that I was either going to be miserable and treat my mom just as miserably and be a very bitter girl when she was gone, or I could put myself in therapy and forgive her.

My dad found me an awesome therapist in the city, an older man who was unlike any other therapist I'd seen previously. He'd never heard of Aerosmith. Or my dad. He looked like a wise old professor, and he listened to classical music. Of course timing is everything. I was ready for help. I was very honest with him. He also asked good, direct questions that hit home, starting with the obvious one: Why was I there?

"My mother is dying and I'm angry and freaking out," I said.

"Why are you angry?" he asked.

"I have hated her my entire life," I said. "At times, I wished that she were dead. And now she's dying."

"You don't think it's because you wished it?" he asked.

"No."

"But you feel guilty?"

"No. I'm just unbelievably pissed off at her."

"Why?"

"For the things she did to me as a kid. For all the complaining she did. And now because she's dying."

"Why are you pissed off at her for dying?"

"Because she never got a chance to live. She never let herself live. She just sat around complaining and wasting time."

"Isn't that her problem?"

"I suppose."

"Why are you making it yours?"

"I'm scared and angry."

"How do you think she's feeling?"

"I don't know."

"Have you asked her?"

"She said she's scared and angry."

"Rightfully so, don't you think?"

"Yes."

"Why else are you angry at her?"

"Because she's not going to be around."

"I thought you hated her. What do you care if you hate her so much?"

"I'm going to miss her."

"Okay," he said. "Now we're getting somewhere . . ."

In early June, I got my mom and dad to make amends. He had been justifiably angry at her following the publication of her book, her subsequent attempt to include nude photos of him in the paperback edition, and then her effort to sell them online. But Liv, Bebe, and I all teamed up and appealed to him to reconcile with her. We didn't have to try that hard. As he once said, there's a part of him that still loves every woman with whom he's ever been seriously involved, including my mom.

He was also in a good, forgiving space. In January 2001, Aerosmith had triumphed as the halftime act at Super Bowl XXXV, delivering an over-the-top version of "Walk This Way" with guests Britney Spears, Mary J. Blige, NSync, and Nelly. Two months later, they released their thirteenth album, had a Top 10 hit with "Jaded," and were inducted into the Rock and Roll Hall of Fame.

At my prodding, he and my mom got together for brunch at Balthazar, and then they walked around Soho. Given her condition, she looked terrific. Even her cane, which Keith had made and hammered full of copper, looked cool. Afterward, she laughingly described the afternoon as "the usual Sunday bullshit," but I could tell that she genuinely appreciated the time they spent together. She acknowledged they'd done a lot of healing and recommended not waiting twenty years to patch things up.

"Next time 'round," she said with a laugh, "I'll do it immediately."

After that brunch, we moved her into the Gramercy Park Hotel. It was near Beth Israel Medical Center, where she received her chemotherapy and radiation treatments. My dad covered her room, board, and personal care—anything she needed. Medicaid took care of all her medical bills. Keith, who moved into the hotel with my mom, called my dad their "guardian angel."

And he was. But his generosity came with a terribly ironic twist. For her entire adult life, my mom had wanted my dad to take care of her. Now that he was paying for everything,

That was so true. You always have to ask, at what price?

I thought of the warning she'd once given to me: Be careful what you wish for.

In early July, my mom's friends hosted a fund-raiser for her at CBGB's, the famous downtown rock club where she'd spent some of the best times of her life. My mom wore a stylish blazer and a blondish-brown wig. Liv and I sat next to her as she visited with dozens of people, including Bebe; Liv's boyfriend and future husband, Royston Langdon; and former Warhol pals Penny Arcade and Jayne (formerly Wayne) County, whose performance of the Rolling Stones' "Paint It Black" with the band Church of Betty had my mom clapping in her chair.

Throughout the evening, which included a silent auction featuring autographed guitars from both my dad and David Bowie, my mom looked relatively strong. She was all about her friends and the bands. The threads she'd woven throughout her life had come together in a warm, vibrant, appreciative, raucous, and loving tapestry. She had the sense that she was important to people, that she mattered in their lives and of course vice versa. That's really what she'd always craved; more than a name that was

boldface in the columns, she'd wanted a sense that she'd made
real and meaningful connections with people. She just didn't
know it.

That summer was busy. I did shoots for H&M and *Talk* and *People*
magazines, made several trips to Europe, and promoted the release
of *A Little Bit of Lipstick*. As a present for all my hard work, I bought
myself a toy Chihuahua that I named Pig. My mom no longer left
her hotel room. I brought her pot, which alleviated her discom-
fort. Keith was by her side day and night. Friends visited steadily.
Some prayed with her. One led a spiritual healing attended by a
group of her friends.

By September, I was making plans to travel to Europe for an
H&M shoot in the middle of the month. On the morning of September 11, my phone kept ringing. I slept through the first few
calls. I finally got out of bed, went downstairs, and checked my
message machine. It was my friend Rene, screaming, "It's chaos
outside." I thought he meant that he was at the nightclub Chaos.
I didn't get it yet.

Then the phone rang again. It was Liv, who was crying and
freaking out. She told me to look outside, that a plane had flown
into one of the twin towers at the World Trade Center. I turned
on the news as the second plane hit the other tower. All I could
do for the next few hours was sit and watch reports on TV and
answer the phone, which kept ringing with either family or friends
calling to talk about what had happened.

Later that morning, the phone went down. Scared, I got
dressed and went outside to see things with my own eyes. I grabbed
my camera and photographed scenes that caught my eye. I saw
people covered in soot. The cops set up barricades and wouldn't
let you past Fourteenth Street unless you lived in the neighborhood. Downtown New York was a place of fear and confusion as
well as heroism and humanity.

I left for Paris a few days later on the first plane allowed out of

JFK. I had a shoot for H&M. Like every other New Yorker, I was still in a state of shock. Before leaving, I spoke to my mom, who was by herself. Keith had something to do and wasn't able to stay with her. She was sad. My heart ached leaving her alone.

"Don't worry about me," she said. "You have to live your life."

THIRTY-THREE

Matching Stars

My mom's cancer advanced steadily. The toll it took on her, as she regressed physically from a self-sufficient forty-eight-year-old to a frail woman in need of significant assistance, was an unsettling thing to watch. In a relatively short time, she went from using a cane to a walker to a wheelchair. There was no question what was going on, only how fast it would happen and whether we could keep her comfortable.

Though I tried not to, I would remember the doctor saying she had eighteen months and then I'd do the math. A clock ticks for all of us. Hers was just louder.

Some days I sat with her, talking and watching TV. There were other days when I had to force myself to stop by for ten minutes, resentful and not even wanting to touch her. There was a handful of occasions when I found myself alone with her—and those were intense. One of those times, she looked at me and said she had to go to the bathroom. She also wanted to shower. I had to help her.

It wasn't one of those beautiful moments people describe having with loved ones toward the end of their lives. Like everything else with us, it was a struggle. She emphasized her need to go. I considered carrying her but couldn't. Both of us cursed the situation—and each other. Finally, I put her on a blanket and tried dragging her, but I couldn't do that either. Fuck!

I stood over her, crying, swearing, and straining, until finally, feeling more like a triumphant wrestler than a daughter helping her sick mother, I got her into the bathroom, undressed, showered, dressed, and back in bed. A day or two later, I was sitting next to her bed when she got up and used her walker to get across the room. My jaw fell open. I felt like I'd been manipulated earlier.

"What the fuck?" I said, wondering if she'd purposely tested me.

She apologized and explained that while she still had very little strength, she didn't want to put either of us through such a traumatic experience again. Neither did I. Nor did I press the issue. The earlier episode may have been her way of testing me, of wanting to feel close to me, or perhaps that I was close to her, so close that I'd actually had to undress and bathe her. If that was the case, fine. Because thinking about it later, something more significant stood out to me, something that I'd carry in me after she was gone. My mom had hated her mother so much she'd run away. Despite feeling similarly, I hadn't run away—and I suspected both of us were better for it.

Like it or not, the two of us were links in a continuum. Funny enough, the couple times when we spoke about death, we did it in the context of staying in touch, with me saying that I wanted her to send me signs when she got on the other side. I asked her to call me on the phone, screw up the pictures in my house, or fuck with something of mine. Just let me know she was there.

My cousin Julia visited frequently, too. When the two of us sat on my mom's bed telling stories about the summers we spent together, my mom lit up, even when the tales we told were about getting high on whipped cream or finishing the booze she and her friends had left on the kitchen counter. One day, as we hung out with her and Keith, my mom suggested that she, Julia, and I get matching tattoos as a way of always remaining together.

"Like this one," my mom said, pointing to the Celtic-like cross she had on her forearm.

I didn't have to think. Neither did my cousin. Both of us said yes. We decided on matching stars. A friend of mine came over and did the work in the room. When I said something about it hurting, my mom jokingly pointed to the vials of pills by her bedside and said she had enough painkillers for everyone in the entire hotel to get a tattoo without feeling any pain.

Later, Keith added some touch-up work (he put a small chain on mine, so it looks like it goes up my arm). I remember watching the way Keith tended to my mom and realized, sadly, that these were her best days—as well as her worst.

After Christmas at my dad's, I picked up a carload of my mom's stuff from her friend's house in upstate New York and brought it back to my apartment. I wanted to go through the things she'd put in storage in case I came across anything that I wanted to ask her about. It was my last chance. My therapist also pointed out that I was looking for ways to connect with and be close to my mom, both in the past and present.

Okay, I wasn't going to deny that. Her stuff filled up my place so much that I felt claustrophobic, though it may have also been the memories crowding me as I let them out of the boxes. She'd packed up everything: eight million books, photographs, clothes, and doodads. When I asked her about a few of the things, she shrugged to let me know she didn't want to deal with the memories or she said she didn't remember. Basically, she had no interest the past anymore. Everything was about the moment.

In early April, I moved into a new place on Eighth Street. I'd had the movers pack up all my shit, plus my mom's, and then I left it stacked up in my new place. I was busy; between my mom fading and a couple jobs that happened at the time, I felt too unsettled to unpack. When I finally saw a window of free time for unpacking, my stepmother Teresa called and asked if I planned on going to L.A. for the MTV Icon tribute to Aerosmith. According to her, it was only the second time MTV had produced an event like this honoring a band. She and my dad were taking Chelsea and Taj. Liv was also attending, she said.

"I just moved into my place," I said. "I literally haven't even spent the night here. Or opened any of the boxes, for that matter. I don't even know where my passport is—or my keys. The movers put *everything* in boxes."

"You have to come," she said. "Everyone's going to be there."

Although I wanted to spend the week unpacking, I signed up for the family trip. I stayed up well past midnight searching through boxes until I found my passport, which I used instead of a driver's license. It turned up in the second-to-last box that I checked. Relieved, I caught a cab to the airport early that morning. By afternoon, I was in L.A., where ironically I was the first of the Tallarico clan to arrive at the venue.

Being at the show was great. Sitting next to Liv and the others in the front row, I was glad that I'd made the trip. I was proud of my dad. There were also four guys sitting right behind us who livened up the time prior to the show with their funny, borderline rude comments. I recognized them from the band Papa Roach. A few months earlier, I'd bought their CD. I didn't even have a stereo at the time. But I'd been so into their single "Last Resort" that I went out and bought one.

I whispered to Liv that their singer, Jacoby Shaddix (formerly Coby Dick), was hot. He had tattoos and eyeliner. I had no idea that he was married and his wife had given birth to a baby boy two weeks earlier. Glancing over my shoulder, I thought the others looked interesting, too, and I searched for a way to make conversation.

My opening came when I overheard them wonder whether there was an after-party and if so, where it was. I turned around and gave the details.

They ignored me.

"I'm not kidding," I said.

They still ignored me. Fine. If they were going to be such dicks, I wasn't going to bother.

After the show, I wanted to go back to the hotel and visit with several friends of mine in L.A., but Liv persuaded me to go with her to the after-party and get some champagne. It was a good move. The party, held under a giant tent next door to the venue, was clearly the place to be in Hollywood. No matter where I looked, I saw someone famous, including Cher, Pink, and Pamela Anderson. Liv and I stood next to my dad, snickering privately as we eavesdropped on Hollywood types and record executives sucking up to him. Then I spied Simon Rex sitting on a couch across the room. I nudged Liv. Look! I reminded her of when he was the hot MTV VJ and naked pictures of him popped up on the Internet.

"He had a giant you-know-what," I said.

She laughed.

"I'm going over to talk to him," I said.

After crossing the crowded space, I got to Simon at an opportune moment: he was by himself. I sat next to him and struck up a conversation. At a point when it seemed like we were hitting it off, I took the very bold, what-the-hell step of telling him where I was staying if he wanted to have fun later that night. He offered some bemused response that meant thanks but no thanks.

That rejection turned out to be fortuitous, as it caused me to look for another place to go, and that's when I looked up and noticed Papa Roach drummer Dave Buckner standing a few feet away. A little over six feet tall and nearly 230 pounds, he didn't stand as much as he loomed. Although not my type, I felt an invisible force pull me to him. It was weird. I walked over to him without even saying good-bye to Simon and began talking to Dave.

I can't remember how we started talking, but it was a friendly conversation about music, the show, and his band Papa Roach. He seemed funny, spiritual (he'd showed me some cool Buddha beads and talked about a large Buddha he had at home), and like a good guy. The whole time we spoke a largish girl stood between us. I thought she was with Dave. He thought that she was my friend. As we exchanged numbers, he leaned forward and whispered, "Do you know her?"

"No, I thought she was with you," he said.

We laughed. Dave said Papa Roach had a show coming up in New York that summer. I told him to him call me when he got into town.

Who knew if he would.

THIRTY-FOUR

Just Kissing

Early that summer, I was getting off a plane at JFK after flying back from a job in London. I'd spent most of the flight sleeping and thinking about a fling I'd had the night before with a handsome guy whom I'd met on the shoot. I wasn't so much thinking about the fling as I was puzzling over why I'd let Mark read some of my poetry, something I'd never permitted—not even with my close friends.

Perhaps I felt safer because I didn't know him, though I suspected the real reason also included a need to share more than my body. I needed a deeper, more lasting and significant connection. That was true in all aspects of my life. My mom's illness was causing me to ask questions about the direction I was headed. While answers didn't magically appear, I sensed that I was past the darkest moments, like the one the previous year in L.A. when I contemplated suicide.

I have to admit that it helped that my therapist had put me on medication. Still, I wondered if I was coming into my own—or even what that meant.

Anyway, as the jet taxied to the gate, I checked my messages and heard a voice that wasn't instantly familiar. Then he said his name, Dave, and I recognized his voice at once. It was Dave from Papa Roach. He said that he was going to be in New York in three days. His band had a show at Jones Beach, and he invited me to be his guest.

If he hadn't also said that I could bring friends, I doubt that I would've gone. Having been away, I wanted to hang out at home. Believe it or not, I still hadn't finished moving into my apartment. But I rounded up a couple friends and we hopped on the Long Island Railroad. When I found Dave, the band Incubus was midway through their set, and he took me to watch from the side of the stage.

He grabbed ahold of my hand as we walked through the crowd. I noticed that my hand was kid-sized in his bearlike grip, and it felt good. The way he led me around also made me feel safe. I didn't realize it until later, but I was looking for that kind of security, given the uncertainty my mom's illness injected into my life. But Dave said he had a girlfriend, a fiancée, in fact; that didn't make me feel too comfortable. That's when I pulled my hand from his. I made it quite clear. I didn't want a photo of me hanging out with the Papa Roach guy to show up in a magazine.

But it was also clear that we'd hit it off. There was something going on between us.

The band had lined up a bunch of festival gigs in the Northeast, and they were based out of New York City, so Dave and I saw a lot of each other. If we weren't hanging out, we were talking to each other on the phone or texting. I enjoyed having a new friend, which was the way I thought of him. But Dave made it quite clear that he wanted more than friendship. He wanted benefits, too.

In a way, he was like my dad had been twenty-two years earlier when he scratched at my mom's hotel room door. Dave thought music was his way to get closer to me. Once, when I'd gone to visit him at one of the nearby festivals, we were hanging around the backstage area, near their tour bus, which he wanted to show me. He was heavily into Bob Dylan and pushed me to get on the bus where we could get cozy and listen to whatever Dylan gem he'd recently discovered. I refused.

"I know what happens in the back of the bus," I said.

"What do you mean?" he asked.

"I don't know what kind of girls you're used to, but I don't go in the back of the bus."

"What do you mean?"

"Hey, I was almost born in the back of the bus. I grew up hearing about the back of the bus. My dad helped write the rule book for the back of the bus . . ."

The one time I followed him back there, Dave was in my face the whole time, trying every which way he could to make out with me. Because of his girlfriend, I said no. But I felt my resistance weakening. His persistence was wearing me down. A couple days later, at another gig, we found ourselves talking alone on a sofa in a private area backstage, and we kissed for the first time.

Oh God, I thought, *here we go.* Several more make-out sessions followed that week. It was just kissing. We didn't go further.

I wanted to stay friends. It seemed possible. The band was leaving the East Coast. The night before they headed back west, Dave and I went to an Incubus party. After several hours there, we ended up in his hotel room, telling each other that we were tired and wanted to watch TV rather than party, but we made out as soon as we got to the room. It was part of saying good-bye.

We stayed up late and at some point we fell asleep in each other's arms, clothed. It was only for a couple hours. I was mortified the next morning when I walked through the hotel lobby and the rest of the band saw me as they waited to check out. I knew they thought I'd screwed Dave. I had the urge to tell each one of them that nothing had happened. I didn't. But God knows what Dave told them.

Over the next month, Dave e-mailed me daily. One night he called from Mexico and said he'd bought me a present. Why was he doing that when we were just friends? Another night he called and said he'd thought about me through the band's entire show. A compliment, I thought, but what was going on? I thought about

Dave, too, but I didn't know if I thought about him because I had strong feelings for him or because he was injecting himself into my life.

I was really confused and conflicted when Dave begged me to meet him in Idaho, where the band was playing their last show before taking two weeks off, which meant he'd be home and unable to speak to me because of his girlfriend. Going back to her freaked him out, he said. It freaked me out more.

"I really want you to come to Idaho," he said.

"I don't know," I said.

"I'm buying you a ticket," he said.

"Isn't it going to look weird when you buy a plane ticket?" I asked. "What's your girlfriend going to say about that eight-hundred-dollar charge?"

"Don't worry, I'm going to do it on the band account," he said. "Someone else in the band did that. It was fine."

"Oh, so I'm *that* girl," I said. "I'm a fucking groupie girl you're flying out? No thanks."

"It's not like that," he said. "You don't get it."

I did get it—and that was the problem. I told Dave that I didn't want to be the girl who was flown out. Nor did I want to get involved with a guy who had a girlfriend. She was more than a girlfriend. She was a fiancée. I wasn't into skulking and cheating. Long conversations about his relationship ensued. It was the first time we'd addressed his relationship directly, thoroughly, and honestly. Though they'd been together for five years, Dave swore it was on its last legs. Despite their engagement, he said that they weren't ever going to get married.

"Then break up," I said.

"You don't understand," he said. "It's not that easy."

"It's not supposed to be easy," I said.

"I really want to be with you," he said. "I really want you to come to Idaho."

"I need to know that you're breaking up with her. Not just saying you will. Actually doing it."

"I will."

After those talks, our bond grew more intimate and intense. I kept asking myself what I was getting into. I was starting to fall in love with him, and yet he was engaged. Inevitably, I agreed to go to Idaho. We felt like we needed each other as we went through major life episodes. He was breaking up with his lady, and I was, in a sense, breaking up with my mom.

Upon my arrival in Idaho, I planned to get a cab at the airport and meet Dave at the hotel. Before going to the baggage claim, I paused in the terminal to call Dave and let him know that I'd arrived. As I got out my cell phone, I felt a strong presence behind me. I turned and there was Dave, grinning. A moment later, I was in his arms, beginning the weekend when I dropped my guard and let myself fall in love.

Why do you fall in love? In addition to all the other factors, from compatibility to attraction to timing, I liked Dave's size. Though I never thought about myself in similar terms, in reality I was a big girl and I enjoyed that he was bigger and stronger. We fit together. The two days went by in a blur. Everything was perfect. Then it was over. The band was scheduled to leave before my flight, which was later in the day. As soon as Dave said good-bye and left our hotel room, I burst into tears.

Two minutes later, he walked back to the room. We hugged and cried, not wanting to let go. It was straight out of a movie—a complicated romance.

I'd told my mom about Dave shortly after I first met him in L.A., but she had no memory of that when I saw her again after returning home from Idaho. She was in bed, swollen from medication, and on painkillers. Doctors had given her eighteen months, and she was in month fifteen. We had no idea how much longer she'd last.

I fantasized about telling her the situation with Dave and getting a sense of what I should do. I'd seen that on TV and in movies like *Terms of Endearment*. Family members go to their dying parents for truths about life and love, knowing that with their days numbered, people get rid of all the bullshit in life and are able to see what really matters.

My mom was propped up on two pillows. I got on the bed next to her. A friend of hers sat in a chair in the corner. After spilling my guts, I said, "So, do you think he's the one?"

"I don't know," she said.

I hid my disappointment. That wasn't what happened in the movies. I wanted her to say something profound. I kept asking her the question.

"What do you think? Is he the one?"

Over and over I asked—to the point where she snapped at me.

"I told you, I don't fucking know."

Her friend came over and put her arm around me. She was a very religious woman. She offered a gentle, earnest smile.

"Lately, your mother and I have been praying for you," she said.

"You have?" I asked.

"We've been praying that someone will come along and take care of you the way your mom always did."

I can still see myself rolling my eyes. What was she talking about? What were they praying about? How delusional were they?

THIRTY-FIVE

Lesson Learned

Walking into her hotel room, I was struck by the sight of my mom. She was in bed with her eyes closed, lying in a state between sleep and grogginess. Often cold, she was under a couple layers of blankets. Cups and bottles of pills crowded the top of her night table. I was struck by the thought that she was like a sick infant.

Interesting thing. When I visited her every day, I didn't notice the deterioration as much. It seemed gradual. But having been gone and not seen her for five days, the change seemed more marked, and it shook me. The clock seemed to tick louder. I said something about it to Keith, who patted her leg and assured me that she was comfortable. I sat down and chatted with Keith and a friend of my mom's who was there. Another friend of hers also stopped by and left.

After a while, my mom opened her eyes, nodded at a question, and added a couple words to the conversation later on. She was weak but not out of it. When up to it, she was still strong enough to talk. But she was in her own stream of consciousness, agitated sometimes, calm at other times, clearly going through a panoply of emotions as if reacting to a private review of her life.

On my most recent visits, she'd taken to apologizing over and over—sometimes about specifics, though often it was a general apology. Even when I asked her about Dave, she replied, "I'm sorry." One day I brought up my dad. I told her that she needed to forgive him and, though I didn't say it, in the process release herself from so much anger.

"Look at everything he's doing for you now," I said.

It was true, and she knew it. Everyone in the family had rallied during her illness. The invisible thread had been pulled, and all of us, from Bebe and Liv to my dad to Mom's old friends to my cousin Julia and me, had come together in our own way and let her know that she was important in our lives and loved.

We weren't a typical family, but I saw—and felt—that in a time of seriousness we were a family.

"He's not a bad person, not the way you always made him out," I continued.

My mom took my hand and squeezed it.

"I'll forgive him for you," she said.

"No, if you're going to forgive him," I said, "do it for yourself."

"You're so fucking stubborn," she said. "And smart."

"Hey, I learned everything I know from you," I said.

She smiled.

"By not listening and doing the opposite," she said.

During the last months of her life, she cried nearly all the time. It was impossible to know why. I don't think she knew. Perhaps she was going through the stages of death, working toward some sort of acceptance. All of us were. I cried my share of tears, too. I was sad at losing her, sad for the time she'd wasted being angry, sad at what she was going to miss.

There are those who believe that each of us is here to learn specific lessons and we don't pass until we learn them, even if it's right at the end. My mom was a good example of that. When she met Keith, she learned about love—about letting herself fall in love with someone who loved her back, not because they were famous, rich, or any of the other things that had always been important to her.

And good for her. Keith brought love into her life before it was too late. He was amazing throughout her illness, and he rose to new levels in her final weeks. He fed and cleaned her, and then, when she was in severe pain and wavered in and out of consciousness, he simply hugged and kissed her and, as he said, "let her know that she's loved."

She knew that. One day her friend, author and spiritual healer Kathy Freston, led a prayer and meditation session where her friends gathered and gave her love. And then on August 28, something truly special took place. Keith and my mom got married in her room. Kathy officiated, as Jane Holzer, Patti D'Arbanville, and other friends surrounded my mom, whose pale face was wet from tears.

I'm convinced she would've gone sooner if not for Keith providing her with a reason to live. In her own way, she was a beautiful bride.

By then, we knew she was going to pass soon. Sometimes she opened her eyes and revealed a glimmer of awareness, as if she were looking at us from a distance. Otherwise she slept most of the time. Keith and some of her friends sat with her. They held her hand, burned candles and incense, and did their best to make her transition loving, spiritual, and peaceful.

The doctors said it could be any day. I spent my last moments with her sitting beside her bed as she slept, holding her hand and saying good-bye. There was no point anymore in rehashing the past. I told her that I loved her.

I may not have liked her, but I did love her. And I would continue to learn from her.

> At that point, the only thing that mattered between my mom and me were those three words. I love you.

"Watch over me," I said. "And I'll keep my eyes open for you."

I stayed with her a while longer. If she couldn't hear me, I hoped she could at least feel the flow of energy from my hand to hers. Finally, I kissed her cheek and let go of her hand. It was a real letting go, too.

When I left her room, I headed to the airport to join Dave and Papa Roach on the road in Atlanta. I didn't want to be in town when she died. I didn't want to be the one they called. Keith was there, and that seemed the way it should be.

I was set to fly home following Papa Roach's show in Atlanta, but when I didn't hear from Keith, I continued on to Chicago, the band's next stop. It was there, at nine a.m. on September 7, that my phone rang. It was my dad.

"Mommy died," he said.

Silence.

Then I cried.

"Oh," I said.

"Keith called me."

"At least she's not suffering anymore."

"I know."

I made reservations on the next flight to New York, but I had a wait. Dave consoled me through the afternoon. I went with him to Papa Roach's sound check, where, instead of the tune the band normally played, they ran through "Walking Through Barbed Wire," a sad song that caused me to burst into tears as I heard the words "It's time to say good-bye to you" echo through the venue. I ran out outside, thinking, *Why'd they play that one?*

Later, I found out that Dave had chosen that song. He thought it would be good for me. It wasn't.

My mom's body was viewed at the Frank E. Campbell funeral chapel next door to our old apartment on Eighty-first and Madison, where years earlier she'd told me about the city's elite who'd been eulogized at the stately funeral parlor. There was also a service at St. Ignatius Loyola, the church on Eighty-fourth and Park.

All of her friends and mine showed up. Stepping to the pulpit, Keith scatted a tune that echoed through the large church. My mom would've loved the weirdness of it. I was moved by the service and the stories her friends told. The strange part was that on entering the church, I turned off my cell phone. I remember shutting it off because I'd been fighting with Dave, who was on the road, wasted, and no support when I needed it, and I didn't want him calling me back.

Yet my phone rang several times throughout the service. The first time I thought that I might have forgotten to shut it down. But no, it was off. I double-checked. Then it rang again.

My cousin Julia gave me a look. I whispered that I'd turned it off. It was like we were naughty little girls again. But then it hit me. About a month earlier, I'd asked my mom to give me a sign after she'd crossed over. I'd heard that electronics sometimes behave strangely after someone dies, serving as conduits for the dead. I didn't know whether to believe it. But when my phone rang again, I said, "What the fuck?" and almost burst out laughing.

I knew it was my mom.

"Stop it," I said, looking up. "Not now."

Before leaving the church, one of her friends began telling me some stories about my mom. She knew we'd had a troubled relationship, but she wanted to make sure that I knew my mom loved me.

"I know," I said.

She put her arms around me and drew me close.

"You have to live for her now," she said.

That was partly correct. I had to live—but not for her. I had to do all the things my mom never did, all the things I was supposed to do, and learn all the lessons I needed to learn, but I had to do them for me. As a kid, I learned to do the opposite of whatever my mom did. Since she liked ketchup, I learned to like mustard. As an adult, though, it wasn't that simple. I had to learn from her and make sure that I didn't repeat her mistakes.

It would take a lot of self-awareness, because no matter how much I didn't want to admit it, we shared many similarities. Both of us were rebellious. She'd burned herself as a kid, and I cut myself. Her first husband was a rocker named David. I was in love with a rocker named Dave. The list went on. But I didn't have to repeat her mistakes as long as I was aware of the decisions I made and the ways I made them. I would live for her in the sense that I wouldn't let myself be miserable. But I would face life, the good and the bad, and deal with adversity rather than run or complain.

The end of her life became a declaration for the rest of mine. I was going to get the best of life. I'd take her along for the ride.

My mom was cremated. Picking up her ashes, I was surprised by the weight. They were in a black plastic box that felt like it weighed about twenty-five pounds. I knew it was macabre, but I looked inside. It was like sand, with fragments of bone visible against the finer grain. I didn't know what to think; that was my mom.

We divided her ashes into four parts. Keith and one of my mom's friends got a scoop each, and so did my cousin and me. I decided to take my share of her ashes back home—to her original home—in Santa Monica, where I planned to drop them in the ocean. She was a Pisces; it made sense to put her in the water. My friend Amanda arranged for a boat, and Dave came down from Sacramento. We took the boat far off the coast, dropped a rock Dave's mother had painted with the word HOPE, and then scattered the ashes and a bouquet of flowers into the ocean.

We stood at the rail and watched the ashes and the flowers clump together and drift away in the current. Floating on the surface, they took the shape of an angel. We watched for a long time. I didn't know what the ashes were supposed to do, but they never spread out or sank. Instead the angel shape drifted north.

"Look," I said. "She's not giving up. She's swimming out to Malibu to find some rich lawyer or doctor on a yacht."

• • •

After I got back to New York, I felt like going to Sunapee. Julia went with me. We made a road trip out of it, driving for two days and spending two days at the old house. We didn't do anything special. The point was just to go there, touch base, and reaffirm that part of my life. My mom may have hated the isolation of living in the sticks, but to me that was home. It felt good being there.

Late that first afternoon, I walked to the end of the pier and looked into the water, hoping to catch a glimpse of my mom's purple shoe, the one Julia and I used to dive for every summer. It had been down there since we moved. The water wasn't really warm enough to swim in, but had I wanted to, I could've dived in, flailed around, and found it. But it seemed fitting to leave it in the water, along with that part of my life.

That night Julia and I reminisced about my mom and the past. We laughed and cried in equal measures. Being in that house under such circumstances put me in a mood where I needed to share feelings about life, death, fate, and the shit you can't predict or plan for. Why did my mom get brain cancer?

"She smoked," Julia said. "Shit happens."

"Yeah, but I think it was all the stuff she kept inside her," I said. "Emotional toxins from never dealing with her anger, never moving past it."

I want to believe life is not for nothing. There has to be meaning. There have to be lessons that we're supposed to learn. But no one hands them to you. It's up to us to find them and figure them out. Before dying, my mom was able to learn that she was worth loving again. As for me, I was falling for Dave. All I wanted was marriage and children, the two things I grew up without, and I would end up getting exactly what I wanted, married and pregnant.

Then it blew up in my face and it was as if I could hear my mom's prophetic words: Be careful what you wish for.

THIRTY-SIX

The M-Word

I made it clear to Dave. I wanted to be with him, but not if he was still engaged or involved with another woman.

If he was as unhappy in his relationship as he professed, he had to do something about it, and soon after my mom's passing he broke off their engagement. According to him, he needed more time to end their five-year relationship. But he claimed to be in the process of it. But then his girlfriend found love letters that I'd written in his luggage, and suddenly it was clear that he hadn't told her about me.

The shit hit the fan. After discovering the letters, Dave's ex called up the Papa Roach singer's wife and went ballistic. Then I heard from Dave, who made it seem he was neck-deep in crisis and wanted my sympathy and support.

"She knows about you," he said.

"I hope so," I said. "You were supposed to have told her that you were breaking up and had met someone else."

"You don't get it," he said. "She found love letters you wrote. She knows about you. She knows about us. She's hugely pissed."

"I'm sure," I said. "You obviously haven't told her anything or everything."

"I'm on my way home to deal with it," he said.

He made me a co-conspirator in his breakup rather than take on the responsibility by himself. I didn't like that, but I could see few options other than to wait anxiously by the phone for details. We burned up many T-Mobile minutes between New York and Sacramento during the three months it took him to break up. I hated the way he dragged it out. I like to deal with relationship issues as soon as they come up. If you're unhappy, figure out why. Don't accept unhappiness as the norm.

I wish I had taken my own advice. But I overlooked the frustration I felt as he drew out his breakup because I was so wrapped up in the path he provided to a new life following my mom's passing. Looking back, he was using me similarly as a way to get out of a relationship that wasn't working.

Just before Christmas 2002, his girlfriend finally moved out. It was the present both of us wanted. I flew to Sacramento afterward and we spent New Year's together. We partied hard to avoid the fact that things felt weird and uncertain, like the ground after an earthquake, and we plotted the fun we were going to have together in 2003. And we did. In mid-January, Papa Roach hit the road for their third major tour in as many years, and I went along. They started in Seattle, moved down the coast to Portland, San Francisco, and Los Angeles, and then headed into Texas and Florida.

Dave and I seemed to cover just as much ground. On the road, we had no emotional baggage, no ghosts from a previous life, no rules. We were like actors falling in love on a movie set. In that vacuum-sealed world of long bus rides, sound checks, shows, and then a new city, it was impossible to separate reality from fantasy. As a little girl, Julia and I had played rock wives, pretending to watch our husbands onstage and then throwing parties after the show. I laughed at the memory as I lived that life, minus the wedding ring, of course.

I liked the social part of meeting young guys in rising bands that I listened to. I also liked that they weren't my dad's contemporaries. I was clearly in a chapter of my life that was a result of my own hard work, not one handed to me because my last name was Tyler. Similarly, Dave had his own money and independence. Unlike most of the guys I'd dated in the past, I didn't have to pay for everything. He impressed me as serious, spiritual, earthy, and sensitive, especially when he focused his attention on me.

Looking back, there were little moments on the road when guys in the band, their ladies, or several people who worked for Papa Roach sidled up to me and asked how things were going with Dave. When I said things were great, they nodded warily, said "good," or expressed surprise. After several months on the road, some of those questions turned into outright warnings. One guy said that Dave was a handful. Another elaborated on that, explaining that he hadn't shown me the real Dave.

The real Dave? I hadn't seen any kind of unusual behavior. We were as close, if not closer, than ever. I chalked those comments up to tension between bandmates and looked forward to the end of summer when the band would take a break and Dave and I would hunker down, just the two of us, in Sacramento.

Dave lived in a two-story, four-bedroom home in a nice neighborhood of midsized homes about five minutes outside of Sacramento's airport. Like me, he made his home a sanctuary, a comfortable place where he could shut out the world. He had two living rooms, one with a large Buddha statue and a little waterfall and another one for kicking back in front of the TV with beers and a bong.

The walls were painted a relaxing cream color, but there was nothing on them and not much in the way of furniture. Normally I would've undertaken the challenge of making the place warm and comfortable, but we decided to start fresh by finding a new home that would be ours.

At the end of the summer, we found a house across the street from where the band's singer, Jacoby, lived. The house was expensive, but Dave and I decided to make an offer. Someone else made an offer at the same time, and we got into a bidding war. I felt as if my life suddenly got more intense and serious. Dave and I weren't even engaged, and yet we were talking about spending large sums of money and taking on a thirty-year mortgage.

Late one afternoon, after a meeting with our Realtor, Dave and I stood in the kitchen strategizing about whether to make another bid on the house we wanted when he shook his head, as if feeling the same quickening of events that had left me breathless. But instead of slowing down, he sent us hurtling forward at warp speed.

"If we're going to buy a house, we should just get married or something," he said.

What?

He'd just said the M-word. I had thought about marriage, but not in such a short time frame. It was one of the few times in my life that I can remember being speechless. Dave interpreted that delay as a hesitancy on my part.

"Well, I don't know," he said. "Do you want to?"

"I don't know," I replied. "Do *you* want to?"

"Why not."

There were dozens of reasons why not. But it wasn't said as a question.

"Me too," I said.

"Then I guess we're engaged," Dave said, hugging me.

"Congratulations," I said, kissing him.

I'd always promised my little sister Chelsea that she'd be the first to know if I ever got engaged, so I broke the news to her after tracking her down at Space Camp. She put me on speakerphone and screamed. Then I called my dad and Teresa and Liv, as Dave filled in his side of the family. In lieu of expensive rings, Dave and I got matching tattoos (two stars—one blue, the other red) on our ring fingers.

We ended up losing the bid on the house, but it seemed for the best since Papa Roach was about to relocate to Los Angeles, where they were going to spend the rest of the year recording a new album. I flew back to New York and spent a whirlwind three days packing all my stuff in boxes, arranging for them to be shipped west, finding a new home for one of my two cats, and then taking the other one and returning to Sacramento.

From the moment I got off the plane, it was like crashing into a wall—except the wall was Dave—and when they exhumed me from the wreckage everything was different. I couldn't put my finger on it, but I quickly found out Dave wasn't the same guy that I'd known for nearly a year. The guy who'd spent all his time and energy trying to impress me and make me love him went into hibernation, and in his place was a bear of a man who came to resemble the "handful" I'd been warned of.

It didn't actually start on the drive to L.A., though that six-hour drive, which immediately followed my six-hour flight, was miserable. We settled into a furnished apartment in Hollywood. Dave went to the studio the next day, and I found myself alone in a strange place without anything to do. Even though I didn't have a driver's license, I spent the next few days driving around town in Dave's car, blasting music and trying to get my bearings.

Pretty soon we developed a routine where the guys worked in the studio all day and then we partied our brains out at night. The paparazzi took our picture outside clubs and restaurants. Dave ate up the publicity—and the unbridled lifestyle. A different Dave emerged. One afternoon, as I straightened up the apartment, I came across some pornography carelessly hidden in Dave's stuff. I'm no prude, but the material was extreme. It made me sick. I didn't say anything either. I didn't want him to know that I'd found it.

Mistake. There was a side to Dave that I didn't know, a side that I wasn't sure if I wanted to know, and yet I was engaged to him. I remember having an aha sort of moment, thinking, *Of course, he's a Gemini—a twin.* I knew the good one, and now I'd met the bad one.

After we first got to know each other, I told him that I'd had a coke problem and didn't do it anymore. Out of respect, he quit doing coke, too—at least when we were together. But through

September and October, his drinking and drug use came to include coke and pills. We fought daily about drugs and his escalating use. And going out. I would need downtime to recoup, and yet his partying was like his drinking. Once he started, he didn't stop.

One night I had to carry him down the hallway, and he weighed more than 250 pounds. It epitomized my struggle with him. Yet I loved Dave. My instinct was to try to fix him. I knew he was out of control, but I didn't think he was *that* out of control, nothing I couldn't handle. Years later, a friend said I was obviously wrong and she pointed out that I may have been trying to repair him as a way of making up for not being able to save my mom.

She may have been right.

THIRTY-SEVEN

I Do, I Do,
I *Think* I Do

At the end of October, Aerosmith had a concert date at the MGM Grand hotel's Garden Arena, in Las Vegas, and Dave and I decided to go see them. My dad wasn't a fan of Dave. When I introduced them, Dave had worn a baseball hat that said LIVE FAST DIE YOUNG. Referencing it, Dad asked Dave what drugs he'd done. Dave boasted of having done everything. Later, in private, my dad had let me know that he thought Dave needed to grow up and get his shit together.

I don't think he'd changed his mind when we arrived in Vegas, along with Papa Roach's road manager, Richard, and Richard's roommate, Darrin. But Dave and I had been together for more than a year, and while visiting backstage before the show, I told my dad how we'd talked on the long drive about getting married at one of the little quickie wedding chapels in town.

"Don't do that," my dad said. "You guys should get married onstage tonight."

Dave and I laughed.

"What are you talking about?" I said.

"Yeah, just get married onstage," he said. "It's better than a chapel."

The idea, so whacked it made sense, took on a life of its own. Aerosmith's road manager made some calls, found out it was possible, and about twenty minutes before the show someone got ahold of a local judge who said he could do it. He arrived halfway through the show. Joe Perry had asked Dave and me to pick the spot in the show where we wanted to get married. I chose a place during the encore. Dave and I then watched the show from the side of the stage, drinking and holding on to each other nervously, laughing, kissing, and counting down the songs with growing anticipation.

When Aerosmith reached the point in the show, after playing "Cryin'," my dad walked to the front of the stage and said, "Hey, Las Vegas, I've got a question for you." There was quiet. "My daughter Mia wants to get married tonight." Cheers. "Can I get a witness?" The audience went insane.

That was our cue. Dave and I walked onstage, followed by the judge, who looked nervous as he stared at the packed arena of cheering fans. My dad quieted them down and then handed the microphone to the judge. It was a basic ceremony with traditional vows, except for the thirty thousand people watching and cheering. After I said, "I do," the roar of the crowd was so loud that we couldn't hear anything on the stage. I put my finger to my lips. Suddenly they went quiet.

Whoa! That was power, and I got a big charge from it. I'd spent my whole life watching my dad do that sort of thing, and for a split second I looked at him with a newfound appreciation and, yes, even envy. But there was no time for such reverie. I was in the midst of finishing my wedding vows. Dave said his "I do," we kissed, and all of a sudden we were married. I threw my bouquet—flowers from a vase backstage that a roadie wrapped in gaffer's tape—into the crowd. Everyone cheered and then Aerosmith went into the song "Amazing." And it was.

• • •

Around one or two in the morning that night, Dave, Richard, Darrin, and I went to the Clark County Courthouse to fill out the paperwork needed to make our marriage legal. There, we had yet another ceremony, the quickie version we'd talked about in the car. Richard served as Dave's best man and Darren was my maid of honor. Before completing our vows, the courthouse judge marrying us told Dave and me that we could have one more kiss before we were married.

Thanks to a combination of booze, excitement, and fatigue, I turned around to kiss Darrin. Hey, one more kiss to someone else didn't seem like a bad idea to me.

"What are you doing?" Dave asked, grabbing my arm and gently yanking me away from his friend.

"I thought he meant we could kiss someone else," I said.

In February 2004, Dave and I got married for a third time in Sacramento. To pacify all of our family and friends who called angry at us for marrying without them, we threw the kind of blowout everyone wanted. It was a black-and-burgundy-themed party, but black and blue would've been more appropriate. The days leading up to it were tense and un-wedding-like, especially as my New York friends arrived and I started to entertain at the house.

One night, following dinner, I took my friend Sean upstairs to show him the wedding present that I'd bought Dave. As he looked at it, I heard Dave's voice from downstairs. He wondered where I was. The tone of his voice made me tense. It was like a Pavlovian reaction. Sean saw the change in me and asked if something was wrong. I said no, but that was a lie.

Bracing myself as the two of us went back downstairs, I searched the room for Dave and when I caught sight of him, I silently said, "Uh-oh," because I could tell by the look on his face that he was pissed.

"What were you doing with *him?*" he asked me, not caring that Sean could hear.

"Nothing," I said. "Showing him something."

"Yeah? What were you showing him?"

Fearing that we'd been fooling around, Dave freaked out. I was blown away by his irrationality, insecurity, and anger. He didn't believe my explanation about having bought a present for him, and he kept up his tantrum until I showed him. Then he sulked because he hadn't known to get me a present. He ruined the surprise. He reminded me of when my mom had screamed, "I am fucking Santa Claus!"

The next afternoon was the wedding rehearsal. I don't know if my dad tried to send me a message, but as he walked me down the aisle, he whispered that he'd heard DreamWorks had just dropped Papa Roach from the label. In retrospect, I wondered if he was really asking, "Are you sure?"

Not that it mattered. We were already married. And later that night Dave and I, wearing variations of burgundy and black (I chose a black and burgundy corset with my boobs spilling out) did it again. Dave's mother, a psychic who claimed that she'd worked for the U.S. military during the first Gulf War, performed a New Age ceremony that lasted forty-five minutes and included various Native American blessings and chants. The ceremony lasted so long that I wonder if she stacked one blessing on top of another to ward off a bad premonition.

As we exchanged vows for the third time, I thought of how they had changed from "I do" to "I *think* I do." As I think back on it now, his mother may as well have said, "I now pronounce you Dumb and Dumber." But I had to learn that for myself.

In the weeks and months that followed, we continued to fight. Some things seemed petty. Like when we went out for dinner, he chose restaurants with a buffet, and coming from New York, I preferred nicer establishments—not fancy, just places with a menu. Other things were deeper. In lieu of the designer clothes I wore in New York, I put on baggy T-shirts and jeans. I also quit doing my hair and makeup. Much later, I'd remember my mom commenting that she'd stopped wearing her leopard pants after we moved to Sunapee from New York City because people there didn't dress like that. I felt the same way about Dave's crowd in Sacramento. I went from a world of high fashion to one where most people were just high. I may never have thought about such changes in my appearance except that Dave criticized me for not having any style.

The irony of that comment was a bitter pill. I'd put my modeling career on hold to spend time with him. I could've had all the style I wanted. But he had in mind a different style, one that he liked. He wanted me to dye my hair blond-brown and get my nails done in the style of the girls he admired in Sacramento. I acquiesced on the nails but not the hair. Without realizing it, I also gained thirty pounds. Essentially I wasn't being me. I was conforming to a life and a lifestyle that didn't feel right.

Following our wedding, the band basically spent the next eighteen months on tour, with time off every three months. I visited on and off through the spring, but the fun from the early days was gone. We fought about everything from what I wore to what we ate to how much he partied. Fighting became a part of our routine, the way we spoke to each other when we weren't trying to figure out why we fought or apologizing for having fought.

I found myself preferring to stay in Sacramento and hang out with my new best friend Jen Sand, a spunky businesswoman in San Francisco. We'd met at a mutual friend's birthday party. Six years older than me, she reminded me of the dynamo my mom could've been if she'd moved on with her life.

Her visits to Sacramento provided me with necessary relief. We lay out by the pool, read all the rag mags, played games in the pool, gossiped, and barbecued. Sometimes my old friend Gillian, who'd also moved to San Francisco, joined us. I also had my friend Allie. I appreciated—no, in fact, I *needed*—the female bonding. It was like being a kid again, when Julia and I spent all day playing in the lake.

Julia was the one person to whom I confided the worst parts of my marriage, my struggle to make it work. One day, after Dave and I had been partying too hard and too long, I blew. He was about to go back on tour with Papa Roach for the summer, and I was unhappy with myself for the way I'd been behaving. We got in a big fight, and I stormed out of the house and went for a drive.

When I returned, I found Dave in the fetal position on the bedroom floor, crying in a semi-awake semi-asleep state of mind. Leaving him alone, I went downstairs, where I noticed the blinking light on the answering machine, indicating a message. I hit the Play button and listened. It was Dave's mom, calling to speak to me and saying that the fight wasn't Dave's fault. According to her, it had been my mom, channeling herself through him because she was jealous of my relationship with my father.

I didn't know how to react. I called Jen and said, "You will not believe the shit I listened to just now."

Like me, she didn't know whether to react with shock, disbelief, nervous laughter, or all of the above.

"What are you going to do about it?" she asked.

"I don't know," I said. "Probably nothing. I'll just let it pass and wait for him to get in a better mood."

There was another reason I wasn't going to do anything. But I wasn't ready to share that with anyone, not even my closest friend.

THIRTY-EIGHT

Careful What You Wish For

Since we'd met nearly two years earlier, I'd made it clear to Dave umpteen times that I didn't want to do cocaine. I'd been open about my past abuse. I'd told him that coke was the one drug that I knew without a doubt had power over me. It scared me. I feared losing control if I started doing it again. Yet during the summer of 2004 he talked nonstop, if not obsessively, about doing coke and beyond that wanting me to do coke with him, as if it was a personal goal to weaken my resistance until I gave in. He even started doing it in front of me.

Over the Fourth of July weekend, I caved. Dave was home on a weeklong break, and we stayed up for days partying. During that coke-fueled stint we had some of our best and deepest talks, but on the sixth Dave was in Michigan and I was by myself, glad that he and his coke were gone but feeling rotten from the post-coke comedown/hangover. It was as if all the air and water had been sucked out of me—and the human body is like 98 percent water.

However, I feared there was another reason that I felt lousy. My period was late, something that never happened. With all the uncertainty in my life, there was one thing that I could count on for sure since I turned thirteen, and that was getting my period on the day I was supposed to get it. Concerned that I was pregnant—something Dave and I had purposely not avoided for the past six months—I tried to find a gynecologist in Sacramento. It wasn't an easy task. I either had to wait for four months to see a female doctor at Kaiser or I could see a clinician right away.

Neither option appealed to me and the urgency I felt. So I flew to New York and spoke to Liv, who got me in to see her ob-gyn. Relieved when my pee test came back negative, I returned to Sacramento and spent about a week going about my business. Then it was like I ran into a brick wall. One day I couldn't get off the couch. I slept there for three days, waking up on the last day with cramps. I told Dave, who thought it might be a stomach bug, and I agreed, thinking it would pass.

But it didn't. The next day I went to the bathroom and saw that I was bleeding. There were things coming out of me that were unlike anything I'd seen. It was gross. It terrified me. For a moment, I told myself that it was my period and that I was bleeding more heavily than normal because I'd been late, but that was naïve and wishful thinking on my part. When the bleeding continued that day I called the lady doctor who'd seen me in New York in a panic. She found me a local doctor in Sacramento. I called him, described what was happening, and he said, "If you fill up your tampon in an hour—"

"I'm filling it every ten minutes," I interrupted. "Things are coming out of me. It's disgusting."

He asked questions. We spoke for some time.

"It sounds like you're having a miscarriage," he said.

I spent all week rushing back and forth between his office and the toilet. The doctor figured I was about three weeks pregnant. Even though he said there was no explanation for why I had the miscarriage, I blamed myself. It was too coincidental for it to have happened right after I'd done coke. I went into a severe funk. It was the first time in my life when I really wished that I could've called my mom, and I cried my eyes out for days because I didn't have her or anyone else. I was by myself in a town where I really didn't know anyone or even have my own doctors. I felt like crap and thought about how I'd fucked up my chance to have a baby.

Furthermore, I wasn't getting the support I needed from Dave, who was going from city to city and still partying like it was the Fourth of July. All I'd wanted since I married Dave was a family. That's all I wanted, period. I was trying to make up for what I never had growing up. Yet each time I'd think about it, I'd hear my mom cautioning me: Be careful what you wish for.

At the end of July, Dave flew down from Seattle and took me on the road with him. Still weak and bleeding, it felt good to be rescued from the dreary surroundings of home. I rode the bus with him from Seattle to Chico and back home to Sacramento, where we stayed overnight, and then left for San Francisco and Los Angeles, then went up to Santa Cruz, Madera, and Modesto.

I needed care and comfort, but one night in the coastal city of San Luis Obispo Dave indicated that he'd reached his limit in how much he had to offer by telling me that he was thinking about having an affair because I wasn't having sex with him.

What?

We were on the bus as he told me, and not only was I aghast at the insensitivity and self-centeredness of the words coming out of his mouth, I was equally mad at the band's guitarist, who was sitting nearby, listening to the way Dave was treating me, and not saying anything. *How dare he*, I thought. *How dare both of them!*

It was August, and I'd been bleeding nonstop for two and a half months. I was still uncomfortable and in pain. Dave had no idea of the extent. Clearly.

Forget that I was angry, hurt, and disgusted by his comment. Beyond all that, I was shocked. How could you say that to someone you purported to love? How could you behave that way?

All I wanted to do was get away from Dave and the other guys, and that's what happened. Dave and Papa Roach went off to Europe through the middle of October, and I returned to Sacramento, knowing that he was going to cheat on me, that our marriage was doomed, and that because I was a headstrong, stubborn, and stupid Capricorn who didn't believe in walking away from a problem before trying to fix it, I wasn't ready to give up.

Jen, not working at the time, came down from San Francisco and spent time with me by the pool while I recuperated by pouring my heart out to her. Still nursing the emotional pain from the miscarriage and knowing my husband was cheating on me in Europe, I felt lost and alone. I was like a broken-down horse. I remember saying to Jen, "This just isn't me."

In the fall, I accepted an offer to appear on the new VH1 series *Celebrity Fit Club*. It sounded a little odd, but I wasn't working, it was a way for me to lose some of the thirty pounds I'd gained in the past year, it paid decent money, and it gave me an excuse to periodically get out of Sacramento. The cast included Daniel Baldwin, Biz Markie, Kim Coles, Ralphie May, and Wendy "the Snapple Lady" Kaufman.

At the start of the series, I weighed in at 210 pounds and I made it pretty clear that I didn't care about getting thin as much as I wanted to feel healthier. I told the producers about my fragile condition following the miscarriage, but I chose to keep it a private matter rather than make it part of my story line in the show, as they'd suggested.

The show turned out to be a good platform for me. Off-camera, I battled the show's doctor after he went off on me about not losing weight quickly enough and the tension carried over on-screen. I also went off on the trainer, following one of his rants about fat. By the time it wrapped in December of '04, I'd lost twenty pounds. But I still found myself saddled by my problem with Dave, who returned from Europe full of rage. He kicked in doors, broke shoe racks. I spent part of my birthday hiding in the bedroom closet, scared to come out. I remember hearing my family sing "Happy Birthday" to me on the answering machine downstairs.

• • •

In early February, Jen and I finagled tickets to see the New England Patriots play the Philadelphia Eagles in Super Bowl XXXIX in Jacksonville, Florida. Neither of us was a serious football fan, but we were from New England and that provided enough of an excuse for us to get out of Sacramento. Dave, on a weeklong break from Papa Roach's ceaseless touring, came, too, and he behaved like such an idiot, sulking in the backseat of our rental car and acting like a shit-head while we drove around.

It was the first time someone outside of his band and me had seen that side of him, and it left a bad taste in Jen's mouth. From that point on, she gave me the kind of support I needed, which was considerable. I confronted Dave and insisted that he start therapy if he wanted me to stay in the marriage, and he agreed. My former therapist from Promises also flew up and spent several days putting us through intensive couple's therapy as a way of trying to get Dave to see the pain I was in.

In one of those sessions, I brought up an incident that said it all. We'd been at a Papa Roach show when three girls came up to me and said thank you for inspiring them to lose weight and feel better about themselves, itself ironic as I could have told them a thing or two about needing to feel better about myself. After the girls and I had a good talk, David pouted in the backstage area until I dragged the problem out of him. He'd been upset that the girls had paid attention to me.

"How come nobody tells me they love me?" he'd said. "How come it's always about you?"

Dave was back on the road the rest of February and March, and during that stretch our ability to communicate fell apart. Even though we talked five to ten times a day, we argued through most of those conversations. One day Dave called me in a manic state, alternately crying, ranting, and berating me for everything that bothered him. I made marks on a piece of paper every time he called. By the end of the day, I counted eighty-one calls. When he wasn't blaming me for his problems, he was screaming and talking shit about my family. He was clearly annihilated on something, or many things, I don't know. He dug into my most sensitive areas with a surgeon's precision, knowing what points to hit, until I was a sobbing, shaking wreck.

I finally got off the phone at midnight, not that it stopped Dave from calling. I just quit answering it. After a whole day of insanity, I was exhausted, beaten down, and in more pain than I could remember, including my miscarriage, although that had also been brought up in some of the harangues.

I put on the TV, searched the shows on my TiVo, and chose *Intervention*, the gritty A&E series about people confronting their addiction. I had no idea of the subject matter, but within a moment I was riveted by a girl with pink hair named Tamela who introduced herself as an artist, a singer, a dreamer, "a million things," all of which I related to, especially when I heard her say, "I'm a cutter."

Oh my God. They showed her snapping apart a razor blade while saying, "It's been getting so insane lately. I'm getting . . . completely . . . out of control." A moment later, she'd slashed her arm and was dripping blood. The fascination with which I'd started watching quickly turned to desire as I heard her say the things I felt and then saw her do something that I knew provided relief.

I watched as she took the razor apart and popped the sharp little blades out. *Wow*, I thought, *I can't believe I'd never thought to do that.* Except for the first couple times using a compact, I'd always cut myself with knives. But I'd given my knife collection to friends when I moved to Sacramento. I'd wanted to start with a clean slate, no negativity, nothing that reminded me of the painful past.

The girl Tamela was crying intensely as she made the gashes in her arm, and I cried just as insanely watching her do it. After the episode, I went upstairs to the bathroom and rejoined the estimated two million Americans who self-mutilate. Though I hadn't cut myself for years, I couldn't wait to reexperience the sensation. I methodically took apart my little Venus razor. It had three tiny blades. I assiduously found which of the three seemed sharpest and then went to town on my arm.

God, it felt good. It was better than anything I'd ever done with a knife. With my knives, I cut only a few layers of skin. But with the razor blades I went deep, and it created such an intense and satisfying rush. My eyes burned from the tears that ran down my face. My hands were covered in blood. I loved the way it looked. It looked the way I felt.

THIRTY-NINE

Going Solo

One day I'd gone online and found a website where you could order prescription medication without a prescription. I put in an order for a hundred Xanax and a hundred Valiums. I paid something like $80 and forgot about them. About a month later, I brought in the mail and there they were, two little boxes that when I opened them were like manna from heaven. Since things between Dave and me were continuing to escalate, what could numb the strife better than two hundred tranquilizers?

They came in a box wrapped in newspaper that contained another box and more folded paper. The interior paper was Indian or from some foreign country. It looked cool. I remember thinking that I should keep it. But the pills in the two separate vials appeared exactly the same, tiny white pills. While checking them out, I accidentally spilled the two bottles, mixing pills, though, after much time and careful inspection, I separated them as best I could.

Then I guess I was miserable one day and I popped a couple pills to take the edge away. I thought I took two Xanax, but I may have taken one of each, and then I decided to get something to eat. I called my friend Al, a guy whom I'd met through Dave, and asked if he wanted to meet me at Applebee's. He couldn't. A senior at a local college, he was getting ready for class. But as I said something about not having any food at home and intending to ride my bike to Applebee's, he must've heard something in my voice, or, as he later claimed, he heard me slurring my words, and he skipped class, picked me up, and took me to the restaurant.

According to him, I was out of it. As we ate burgers and fries, I talked gibberish, texted stupid things to friends in New York, and spoke loud enough that he hurried me through the meal before I embarrassed myself. For the next couple weeks, I hit those pills pretty regularly, something I knew was not just wrong but a step backward. After years of dealing with my problems and avoiding drugs other than pot, I was back to cutting and taking pills.

"Am I the crazy one?" I asked Jen one night on the phone. "Maybe it's me, like he says it is."

"No, it's not you," she said.

I asked the same question of others who knew both of us, and fortunately they said the same thing. Otherwise I would've gone off the deep end. On Dave's next break, which came in the early spring, I accompanied him to one of his therapy sessions. It was the first time I'd gone with him to his therapist, and I was shocked by what I heard. His therapist recounted all these incidents and issues, and I was like, "No, no, no, that's not true! That's not it!"

I gave Dave an angry look. He hadn't been forthright with his therapist. We left with even more problems. I was pissed off. I hated that I had to drive back in the same car with him. But when it was just the two of us in the car, he asked, "Can I have another chance?"

I let out a sigh. I knew I couldn't do any more to save our marriage. I couldn't do anything more to help Dave. It was time to help myself.

"No," I said. "I'm out of more chances."

There had been a time a short while earlier when I told one of my friends that my life seemed like a Lifetime movie. Indeed, I felt like I'd reached the point where, emotionally beaten and physically drained, I needed to make my escape. But honest to God, as I told Dave that I wasn't going to give him another chance, I didn't know what to say next. Nor did I know what to do when we pulled into our driveway.

I still didn't picture myself walking out on him. Quite frankly, I didn't have an exit strategy. Then we went in the house and out of nowhere Dave looked at me and matter-of-factly said, "Well, we can call the accountant."

The accountant? First of all, the accountant was *his* accountant, not mine. Second, I wasn't ready to have that conversation. I stood there, feeling my head spin. I didn't know how to end a marriage or divvy things up. Dave went ahead and called the accountant, then put me on the line, and together they said we could make it easy and split without lawyers. I was like, no, no fucking way.

Dave started to intimate that I didn't have anything. But I knew about our finances, and the details poured into my head as if I was some kind of actuarial genius. We'd lived mostly off my money, leaving his savings untouched, so at first glance he may have been right. But legally I knew better. I said, "Are you kidding me? What do you think we've lived on?"

"Don't worry," he said. "I'll make sure you're taken care of."

"No," I said. "*I'll* make sure that I'm taken care of."

Dave and I tried to have one last decent night together, but it ended when he threatened to kill me. Fleeing the bedroom, I ran into the guest room and locked the door as he stood outside and hissed, "At least I can say I was married to Steven Tyler's daughter." Things settled down a bit once Dave went back on the road. I then hired a lawyer and started the wheels spinning toward a divorce.

Dave and I spoke and texted constantly by phone. It was strange; we finally shared a common goal. But he partied hard on the road, and it turned him into a Jekyll and Hyde personality, particularly at night, when he would rant and rage. Knowing we'd reached the end, I tuned him out, treating him like an angry child.

Unfortunately we had an adult-sized mess to fix. I was still in the house in early June when he informed me that he wanted me out by the time he returned before the Fourth of July. Two weeks later, he called and said he was going to be back in three days and again he emphasized that he wanted me *out*. Done fighting, I spent those three days packing. Everything that was mine, from furniture to pots and pans, went into storage, and I checked into a Marriott, where I spent the next fifteen days while he was home.

Once back in town, Dave called and asked where I was staying. He told people—and who knows, he may have also believed it—that I'd left him to be with our friend Al, which wasn't true. Dave knew the reasons I'd left him. Oddly, at his Fourth of July barbecue, Dave took Al aside and suggested he get together with me, allegedly saying something like "Then in about a year we can double date."

When Al told me that, I went, huh? It was too weird, and I wondered why Dave had pushed that. However, Al was among those who provided a comforting, supportive voice, checking in on me daily. I also heard that one of the Papa Roach wives had said, upon hearing we'd split, "I'm surprised she lasted so long."

According to court papers, Dave and I separated legally on July 8, 2005. A few days later, he came back from Hawaii and informed me that he'd met someone else. I didn't care to know any of the details, whether he was being truthful or merely trying to make me jealous. I was free—and relieved. My biggest problems were trying to sleep in the crappy, worn-out bed in my hotel room and figuring out what to do next. Friends checked in on me day and night. That was nice. My BlackBerry pinged nonstop, another comfort.

After two or three weeks, I quit trying to figure out my next move. I felt like I was waking up from a coma. My goal was to walk outside, feel the sun shine on my skin, and not feel tense. As I told Jen and Al, after everything I'd been through, I simply wanted to breathe.

A Reason, a Season, or a Lifetime

*People come into your life for a reason, a season, or
a lifetime. When you figure out which one it is, you
will know what to do for each person.*

*When someone is in your life for a REASON . . . it is
usually to meet a need you have expressed. They have
come to assist you through a difficulty, to provide you
with guidance and support, to aid you physically,
emotionally, or spiritually. They may seem like a
godsend, and they are! They are there for the reason
you need them to be.*

*Then, without any wrongdoing on your part, or at an
inconvenient time, this person will say or do something
to bring the relationship to an end.*

Sometimes they die.
Sometimes they walk away.
Sometimes they act up and force you to take a stand.

*What we must realize is that our need has been met, our
desire fulfilled, their work is done. The prayer you
sent up has been answered. And now it is time to move on.*

*When people come into your life for a SEASON . . . it is
because your turn has come to share, grow, or learn.
They bring you an experience of peace, or make you laugh.*

They may teach you something you have never done.
They usually give you an unbelievable amount
of joy. Believe it! It is real! But, only for a season.

LIFETIME relationships teach you lifetime lessons; things
you must build upon in order to have a solid emotional
foundation. Your job is to accept the lesson, love the
person, and put what you have learned to use in all
other relationships and areas of your life. It is said
that love is blind but friendship is clairvoyant.

Author Unknown

Part Five

I used to look in the mirror and feel shame. I look in
the mirror now and absolutely love myself.

—Drew Barrymore

FORTY

Starting Over

After a couple weeks at the Marriott, I leased a furnished apartment in a complex about forty minutes outside of Sacramento. Al helped me get my stuff out of storage. As we unpacked in my new place, I found the two bottles of pills, my Xanax and Valium. I showed them to Al, who cocked his head in disapproval, recounted our episode at the Applebee's, and said, "Throw those out."

Good advice. Without giving it a second thought, I tossed both bottles and said something along the lines of not only didn't I want to take them anymore, I didn't want to feel like I needed them. Al was a big reason why I felt that way. His companionship and caring nurtured me through the tough, lonely times I had getting back on my feet and feeling self-confident again. In October, after more than two months of doing nothing but getting my head together, we stepped beyond the friendship and kissed for the first time.

It actually happened on a dare from Jen one night as the three of us sat around drinking wine. Aware that I had feelings for Al, she took the initiative. He kept his mouth closed, forcing me to make out with his teeth and then stop when I burst out laughing.

He asked for another chance, saying that I'd caught him off guard. Later, we got rid of Jen and made out for two days straight. We didn't have sex. It was about being in each other's arms. I needed to feel a loving, safe connection, and he felt it in him to give that to me.

From there, our romance developed. It felt right. Not even Dave took issue with our relationship as it blossomed. For almost a year, I didn't do anything other than love Al and let him love me. Literally. While he was in school, I hung out and waited for him. I incurred huge bills for my apartment and rental car; I didn't care. It was part of my healing process. His positive energy flowed into me, rejuvenating every part of my being, deep into my tissues, like pure oxygen.

The best part was that we were equals and I didn't have to pretend or watch what I said. We kept things lively by having "step it up" days, special days when we surprised each other by doing something unexpectedly romantic. It could be a bottle of champagne with burgers, or a walk in the woods after it rained. One time I booked a hotel room for the weekend in Monterey. Another time he got a hotel room for the weekend just to get us away from my apartment.

I'll never forget walking in and finding an iPod playing our favorite music, food laid out, and rose petals sprinkled on top of the bed and in the bathtub. We didn't leave the room for forty-eight hours. It was like a dream.

As with any dream, though, reality eventually intruded. After nearly a year together, Al needed to complete his education and think about a career, while I, having maxed out my credit card and dipped significantly into my savings, began to hear a little warning bell in my head go, Uh-oh, what are you going to do next?

That forced me to address a question that was at the core of my immediate situation, everything that happened next, and also my desire not to repeat my mom's mistakes, namely, how do you start over? Having put my career on hold, moved across the country, married and divorced, and spent a boatload of my money, I was truly at that point where I had to figure out how to reinvent my life personally and professionally.

I thought back to my mom and how she bought one self-help book after another but then left them unread. That wasn't going to be me. However, I didn't buy a book. Thanks to my mom, I instinctively knew what *not* to do. I knew starting over wasn't ever easy. There wasn't a magic formula. There were no guarantees of success. But if I didn't do anything, I could be sure of one thing, more misery.

I realized life is a journey in which you prepare as much as possible and then set out with only a vague sense of where to go. There's no map. And really, there's no set destination. It's as author Douglas Adams said: "I seldom end up where I wanted to go, but almost always end up where I needed to be."

That was the tenor of the discussion Al and I had in early 2006. I knew we had to move on, but first I got through the holidays and the start of the new year before dealing with anything as heavy as splitting from a guy who will always be one of my life's greatest loves. That would've been too hard. But May, the heart of spring, seemed like the right time to make a fresh start. Al agreed. After many long, frightening, and tear-filled talks, we didn't break up as much as we agreed to go in different directions and see each other when we could.

I remember sitting by myself after one of those talks, alone in my bedroom, where my eagerness to leave Sacramento and get on with things surged ahead of my actual ability to get going. It was frustrating. Not until February did I finally and officially nix the idea of returning to New York (been there, done that), get my shit together, and move to Los Angeles; I had a few friends there and I liked the idea of trying to make new connections relevant to who I was at the moment.

I was a mix of exhilaration and fear as I sped down Interstate 5, the straight shot through the center of California, with my music blasting and talking on my cell as if I were taking instructions from Thelma and Louise. After finding an apartment near L.A.'s Koreatown, I found myself with an open calendar and few contacts. Before setting up meetings with agents and managers, I straightened out my résumé. I also spent time getting my website in order. It was like arranging my online home.

As I updated the site, I created a niftier website on MySpace. I surprised myself at the energy I poured into it, and what began as a casual bit of housekeeping turned into a creative endeavor that took on a life of its own almost as if it were a reflection of what I was going through at the time, starting my life over, trying to establish roots, and figuring out my identity.

Indeed, the space became a repository for much more than my bio and career highlights. I put up photos, music, and thoughts that had meaning for me. I put myself up on those web pages— not my career but my private ambitions, successes, fears, and failures. Because I didn't know many people in L.A., I had time to work on the site. I remember sitting in my place on a chilly winter night with the sounds of Koreatown filtering up from the sidewalk, everyone appearing to have someplace to go, someone to go to, while I was having one of those moments where I didn't want to party and wished I had someone with whom I could curl up in front of the TV.

I called Al, who promised to visit soon. Then I turned to the computer and checked the messages on my MySpace. Hundreds had piled up without my notice. I was still new to the MySpace world. It seemed as if overnight I had acquired more than a thousand "friends," people who had somehow found my site, whether by accident or by Googling me. I was blown away.

Hours melted away as I read through the messages, most of which were from young women around my age who were struggling with identity issues or going through their own tough times, some of which were similar to mine, though a significant number were more severe. Like Kristen, a twenty-eight-year-old whose e-mail said "she'd come out the other end after more than a decade of hell." She thanked me for being an inspiration to her. I thought, *Me? How?*

She was the younger of two sisters. She'd always worshipped her older sister, Patty, she said. She'd wanted to be just like her. Except her older sister was tall, thin, and athletic, while Kristen described herself as "short, chubby, and not as much of a go-getter." A couple months before her older sister turned sixteen, the two of them were riding their bicycles, talking about how life would be different after Patty got her driver's license, when suddenly a car sped around the corner and smashed into Patty. She died instantly.

Kristen was traumatized, and her family was devastated. In the aftermath, she said, she tried to replace her big sister. She went out for sports teams in school. She wore Patty's old clothes. She slept in her bed. She even ate the food that her sister had liked. But, she wrote, "it backfired on me. As I grew up, I never felt worthy. I never felt like myself. I wondered why it hadn't been me. I felt like it should've been me. She was better than me. I used to stare at the mirror and want to see my sister's reflection instead of mine."

Ten years after the tragedy, she continued to think that way. She said she often thought about suicide. She relied on drugs and alcohol to numb her pain. Relationships were problematic, if not impossible. "I didn't want to get close to anyone," she wrote. "I didn't want to love someone as much as I did my sister and then have them taken away from me. I wouldn't let anyone love me either.

"Mia, can you imagine the pain and loneliness of living like that every day? I hated myself. I hated my life. I was literally haunted by a ghost."

She wrote that the turning point in her life came one night when she was twenty-six and went into a tattoo shop. She wanted a small flower or Buddhist symbol, but after talking to the tattoo artist, she decided to get a tattoo of her sister. She showed the tattoo artist a photo that she carried in her wallet. She said the tattoo took numerous sessions over several months, and she said the pain of getting the tattoo seemed to exorcise the mental pain she'd carried around for sixteen years.

"I spent hours talking to the tattoo artist as he worked on me," she wrote. "Between the pain and the talking, it was like going through therapy, and I was able to leave the darkness. I'm 28 now, and in the last two years I feel like I've started to live my life for the first time since my sister's death. I don't do drugs anymore or drink till I'm obliterated. I haven't found the right guy yet, but I'm finally open to it. Here's my big insight. If I can love myself, some-one else can love me, too."

Over the next few months I received hundreds of messages simi-lar in one way or another to that one. My friends on MySpace multiplied into the many thousands. I spent hours every day on the site, reading and responding to messages. I didn't fully realize what was going on until I read another message from a twenty-four-year-old woman who said she'd been overweight her whole life and made fun of throughout school to the point where she avoided the smallest glimpse of herself in a mirror or store window.

Mia, I read interviews you gave where you talked about feeling good about yourself and not worrying about looking a certain way. I'd heard others say the same thing, but for some reason you hit home. Maybe it's because both of us have tattoos. Anyway, one day I just said screw the self-hatred. I have a job. I have my health. What the fuck does it matter if I'm not skinny? You know? There are people out there with real problems.

I quit feeling sorry for myself and volunteered at a shelter for abused women and children—you know, people with real problems. Guess what? Those women were great. They appreciated me for just being there and showing up and caring

about them. Amazing. They also laughed at my jokes. They
made me feel like I mattered. P.S.—They didn't give a shit
that I didn't look like Jennifer Aniston. Through sheer
accident, I created a whole new me.

Sometime after reading that message it dawned on me that my
MySpace site was actually an extension of the work that I'd done
as a plus-sized model urging girls to worry more about feeling comfortable with themselves than fitting into a size 2. It had uninten-
tionally grown into that from my simple effort to plant stakes in
Los Angeles. Instead of updating a website, I had created a destination where I connected with other people in a meaningful way
and they did the same.

My days took a turn. I woke up and went straight to my computer, something that I still do. I spent hours there. The morning
flew and suddenly it would be afternoon and I wouldn't have
eaten, showered, or changed from my pajamas. But I was doing
work, offering advice, drawing on my own experiences for answers, and helping other people. One day I asked people to let me
post photos of them. A woman sent in a picture of her daughter
who was going into the navy. Another sent in a photo of herself in
jeans I'd recommended. "They make me look like I've lost fifteen
pounds," she wrote. "He-he!" One woman sent a photo that
she'd labeled "I'm not beautiful, but I'm me!" Someone responded,
"You are beautiful." A dark-haired beauty sent a note with her
photo saying her husband of nearly twenty years had walked out
on her. Another chick wrote, "Screw him. He doesn't know what
he's losing."

And so it went, every day a new adventure into listening,
helping, and engaging in a dialogue that took on a life, or should
I say lives, of its own. I started to feel good, needed, and positive
as I made more "friends" and messages poured in from people
thanking me for providing a place where they knew their self-
worth had nothing to do with the bathroom scale, where they felt
understood and less alone. The really interesting if not ironic part

was that I felt the same way. And one day, in a burst of clarity, I remembered those two simple lines I'd read online that I now know came from Scott Ginsberg. They landed in my head as if I'd seen them scrawled in massive type across the side of the building. I ran to my computer and typed them out across my screen and then loaded them onto my blog as a personal declaration:

"Life isn't about finding yourself. It's about creating yourself."

FORTY-ONE

A Premonition

"I don't really know what I want to do. I'm in the process of creating myself."

I was talking to Andrew Lear, a talent manager at The Core. We were meeting in his office, and I laid my cards out on the table. I told him that I was mostly done with my modeling career, that I thought I was onto something with my website, and that I wanted to try working in TV. Because I had little experience, I said that for the next year I'd take every meeting and meet every production executive in town.

And I did. I was in one meeting with a female executive. She was dressed in a business suit, with a pink silk blouse and Gucci shoes. After listening to me, she leaned across the coffee table that separated her chair from me on the sofa, pushed up her sleeve, and showed me an arm that was heavily scarred.

"Me too," she said.

"When was the last time?" I asked.

"Four months ago," she said. "You?"

"Last year," I said. "Not that long ago, but last year. It was when I was breaking up with my ex."

"I was in the process of breaking up when I did it, too," she said.

Not all the meetings were like that, but enough were. A woman in a different meeting asked about my experiences as a plus-sized model. After I spoke for a while, she opened up about her insecurities working in an industry that clearly favored women who fit into smaller sizes. She never felt pretty or sexy, she said. Then there was the producer who showed me his tattoos and ended up telling me that he was two years sober after a longtime heroin addiction.

"I went to Promises," I said.

"I was at Sierra Tucson," he said.

As I sat in traffic between meetings, got lost, tried out for jobs, went to callbacks, heard from Andrew about rejections, got jobs, and went on more meetings, repeating my story to whoever wanted to hear it, I realized that no matter how frustrated I got, it was all part of the larger, ongoing process of creating myself. Everyone I met was doing the same thing, too. No matter the size, all of us are so alike.

"Yeah, you're all nuts," my manager said.

I laughed.

"Sometimes I feel like a heavy metal Dr. Phil," I told him. "And other times I feel like I should be the patient."

Andrew chuckled and said, "Welcome to Hollywood, kid."

It didn't feel like much of a welcome party, but that was mostly because finalizing my divorce took up most of the summer. After signing the papers, I had good, long talks with Jen and Gillian, got a second "freedom flower" tattoo—my first was after I separated from Dave—on the inside of my right wrist, and reaffirmed the lesson I learned by going through those three years and coming out the other end: Don't let people tell you what you're not or who you're supposed to be. Don't let them destroy you. Don't punish yourself for what others have done to you. You're better than them. You're better than you think. You're as good and powerful and strong as you want to be.

"I have to be patient and tough," I said to Jen one night as we talked on the phone. "And keep believing that one day all that pain will be worth it."

"So true," she said.

"Yeah. Someone e-mailed me that phrase from the poet Ovid—and it is so true: 'Be patient and tough, and keep believing that one day all that pain will be worth it.'"

In September, still not entirely sure of what to do and waiting to hear back after auditioning for several parts, and also inspired by my interactions on MySpace, I got the urge to try my hand at writing music and singing. Al, visiting at the time, encouraged me to go for it if I felt the music in me. I laughed; that sounded like a comment out of the movie *Fame*. Of course the music I felt was much more hard-core than singing "what a feeling." But I did feel it inside me.

I mentioned it to a band manager friend of mine named Gary, who I knew through Dave. Without hesitating, Gary said I should meet a guitar player he knew, a guy named Brain, who was also from up north. He thought we'd hit it off creatively.

That night I went with Al and a girlfriend of mine named Gigi to the Rainbow, the famous rock bar on the Sunset Strip. We were standing in the corner, holding drinks, and talking when Gigi spun me around, pointed to a guy, and purred, "He's hot." He wasn't my version of hot. But I love such moments, especially when I'm a little drunk. I stepped toward him and said, "You! Come over here."

He walked over.

"My friend here likes you," I said, gesturing to Gigi.

He laughed, embarrassed, and then looked at me.

"I actually know your friend Gary and your ex Dave," he said.

Instant buzzkill. I made some snarky remark that made him think I was a major bitch and then he went back to his friends. I didn't speak to him or see him the rest of the night. The following day Gary called me.

"I heard you met Brian," he said.

"Who's Brian?" I asked.

"Brian Harrah—the guy I told you to write songs with," he said. "He said he met you at the Rainbow last night."

"*That* was the guy?" I said.

Having got off on the wrong foot, I sent him a message through MySpace. I apologized, and we chatted for a while and compared our taste in music (he liked the Cure and Clutch, and I rattled off a bunch of bands, including Lamb of God). He preferred bands that were more melodic. I was about to go up north for Al's birthday and said we'd talk more when I returned the following week.

When I got back to town, I felt drained and uninspired from a week of not getting along with Al. Both of us realized we'd come to the end of the road in terms of keeping up any pretense of a romantic relationship. It wasn't fair to either of us. I hated arguing or even being annoyed with him. On the night Brian came over to work on songs, he sensed that something was wrong. We were sitting on opposite ends of the sofa in my living room. he was bald and had a cool tattoo of a tree that I kept looking at. I'd been up and down making tea. At first I said nothing was wrong, and then I told him about Al, which was weird. I barely knew Brian and I didn't feel like opening up about something so personal and complicated.

"Come over here and talk to me," he said, patting the cushion closest to him on the sofa.

"What?"

"Come closer," he said. "It's like we're talking long-distance."

Nobody ever told me what to do. I didn't know whether or not I liked that, but it got me thinking about him in a new way as I moved down the couch. He offered advice about Al that night and on subsequent occasions when we met to work. During those writing sessions, we got to know each other. Like me, he'd grown up in New Hampshire, though not close to Sunapee. But at one point when he was in a band, he went to the mall, and in front of the Spencer's there was a huge poster of his band, and next door was a Lane Bryant with a huge photo of me.

"I used to stare at you all the time," he said. "I can remember looking up at your picture. I had a crush on you, I think."

"You think?"

"It was definitely a crush," he said.

"That's weird," I said. "You knew who I was even before you knew I was with Dave."

"It gets better," he said. "I was once at an Aerosmith concert, one of the shows they did with KISS, and I saw you with your dad. I thought, *There's that beautiful girl I've seen on the photo in that store.* I wanted to meet you."

We got along well and worked easily together. After I knew him about two weeks, we started to talk regularly. One day I was talking to him while I drove across town. I was stuck in traffic on Third Street when I made a last-minute turn up La Cienega Boulevard. For some reason, I asked where he was.

"Look straight up out your window," he said.

I was in front of the Beverly Center shopping mall. I stuck my head out the window and stared up at the parking structure. Brian was on the top floor, waving. I laughed. Then I felt the red-hot flash of a premonition. All of a sudden the traffic cleared in front of me and I sped forward. Brian saw my car lurch.

"I have to go," I said abruptly.

"What's the matter?" he asked.

"I just flashed on the future."

"What?"

"I'm going to have babies with you," I said.

I heard a nervous laugh at the other end before hanging up without waiting for a response. Brian had a girlfriend; that was the unnerving part of my premonition. That he laughed was enough for me. He had a good sense of humor, a prerequisite for working with me. I liked that he didn't flinch at the more outlandish things that came out of my mouth. In fact, later he sent me a funny e-mail.

"You said 'babies'?" he wrote. "Does that mean more than one? If so, we'd better write some hit songs."

He came over a few days later to work and said something funny about being ready to make babies. I joked about how I ordinarily liked dark-skinned Latino boys, but his tattoos made up for the fact that he was white. That led us on a tangent about tattoos. As we shared some of the stories about our tattoos, we discovered that both of us felt similarly about the liberating power of body art. You don't get to choose your nose, eye color, or body shape. But by putting art on your body you're making a statement that's 100 percent you.

I told him about some of the messages people had sent me on MySpace. As the holidays approached, the site got even busier. I saw how difficult the season was for people who ached to be loved and accepted. Reading and responding continued to occupy more and more of my time. I remember telling my dad how the site had taken off, explaining that I felt as if I'd found my niche. He was the family's rock star, Liv was the actress, and I got people in touch with their emotions.

There was a similarity between the way his music and my advice were able to help people through tough moments. Like Sue, a nineteen-year-old who wrote me about having been molested as a kid by her alcoholic father after her mother ran off with another dude. In response, she gained a hundred pounds through middle school, feeling, as she wrote, "more worthless than the dirt on the carpet I stared at when my sick father was raping me of my innocence." She continued,

> How do you recover from something like that? I never tried to recover because I didn't want to live. Every day people talked behind my back. I heard them call me fat, ugly, and more. I wish people knew how easily their whispers can be heard and how much they hurt. Eventually, though, I told myself that they didn't bother me. Do you know why? Because I figured they were right.
>
> I'm not going into the ways I tried to hurt myself, but you can guess. The worst part was the way I isolated myself from

the world. I may as well have been in prison—in solitary
confinement.

But then something happened. Last year, when I was 18, I
made a friend. I had to go to the doctor and I started talking to
the nurse. She asked if I wanted to meet for coffee. No one
had ever asked if I wanted to meet for coffee. We had a nice
time and about a week later we met for dinner and a movie.
She didn't see me as a fat, ugly girl and that made me feel less
unlikable.

It's amazing what can happen when you don't feel like
such a horrible loser. I lost 35 pounds just from being with my
friend when in the past I would've been alone and stuffing my
face from being sad and sorry for myself. I'm still a big girl,
and that's okay. I call myself a big girl with an even bigger
personality. I don't know why I'm writing you since I don't
need any advice or have a question. I though maybe you can
share this and it'll give others hope.

Hope.

That word resonated with me. It was such a powerful idea. I
hadn't thought about it as often as I had about other concepts,
like love and connections, but hope was indispensable to a healthy
outlook. Hope gets you out of your room, out of the house, into
the world. People need to feel hope. I needed to feel hope. I realized that my life in Sacramento had lacked hope. But since moving to Los Angeles . . . suddenly I thought of everything I had
going: starting a new career, my website, the connections I'd
made, writing songs, and Brian. I had no idea where I was headed,
but I saw how everything was related, and I saw that I had hope.

FORTY-TWO

Good Looking Out

Over the next few months Brian and I worked on songs. Talking about ideas took us into places that were extremely personal, and as I'd done with him earlier, he started opening up to me about the difficulties and disappointments in his relationship. We talked about things both of us wanted, a discussion that related to the idea of hope that had been on my mind. We flirted—but only up to a point.

Brian was kind of standoffish in that sense. He made it clear that he didn't want to cheat on his girlfriend. However, I knew two things. He wasn't happy with his relationship, and we were getting closer. Then one night we were at my apartment. He'd come over to work on music. We finally kissed. It was exciting and awkward at the same time. Exciting because both of us wanted it so badly and awkward because we shouldn't have done it.

He went home and then very late that night e-mailed me one of those five-question, answer-honestly personality/relationship quizzes you find in magazines and online. Two days later his girlfriend saw it and freaked out. Neither of us wanted that karma to be part of our relationship, so he dealt with the situation. After they broke up, we began dating.

Unlike with Dave, my dad liked Brian from the start. I intro-duced them one night when my dad was in town for a photo shoot with Kelly Clarkson. Tucked into a corner table at a Hollywood sushi restaurant, my dad gave Brian the third degree. Fortunately, I'd warned Brian beforehand. That was the great thing about in-troducing guys to my dad. They thought they were meeting a cool rock star when in reality they were confronted by Robert De Niro in *Meet the Parents* disguised as Aerosmith's lead singer.

"What drugs have you done?" my dad asked.

Brian looked at me (I'd told him to prepare for that question) and then at my dad.

"I'm not going to lie," he said. "I can count on one hand the times I've tried drugs of any kind. Otherwise I don't do 'em. I drink a little."

My dad kept questioning him. Brian held his own. It became comical as my dad asked him about music, his band, and touring, searching hard for a flaw. At one point, my dad, feigning disbelief, leaned across the table and said, "You mean to tell me that you're on the road, women are throwing themselves at you, and you are on the bus playing *video games?*"

He asked in a way that almost made it seem he was disap-pointed in Brian for getting rock and roll wrong. Yet he still turned to me and said, "Mia, he's all right."

That meant a lot.

I felt like we got close pretty quickly, but Brian had trust issues that made him move slower and more cautiously.

Smart, but frustrating. We dated steadily and more seriously until the summer, when the two of us took a three-week trip to Europe. By that time, we had grown very close and our lives had intertwined in an easy and stimulating manner. I loved him, but Brian was hesitant about giving himself to me. He said it was his problem, nothing to do with me. That left me, as I told him many times, few options besides the very frustrating one of waiting for him to figure out his issues.

I decided that Europe was going to make or break us, and it broke us. Throughout the three weeks we were there, he was reserved and standoffish. I felt it in London, Dublin, and Amsterdam. I would ask him why, which caused him to retreat further. I don't think he knew for sure. I think he was also uncomfortable with his own indecisiveness. Once back home, we had the serious talk that both of us knew was inevitable. He admitted that he wasn't ready for a relationship, to which I replied, "If you aren't ready, then let me go."

He looked shocked; no, make that stunned.

"What do you mean?" he said.

"I mean that I need to move on," I said. "I am ready. You aren't. I have to move on."

It was a hard thing to say, but I wasn't going to torture myself over something that I ultimately couldn't have. I didn't know if I was making the right decision, but my inner voice urged me to choose fate rather than frustration. There is nothing as agonizing and lonely as the days following a breakup. But I didn't sink as far as I had in the past. I wouldn't let myself. I didn't want to punish myself. It was quite the opposite, in fact. Older, wiser, more experienced, I drew on the lessons I'd learned. I reached out to those on my website. I reread a blog post on my site from a few months earlier when, during what must have been a prescient moment, I admitted that I didn't have all the answers and asked my network of friends (by then upward of thirty thousand) for suggestions on what they did to get through the tougher moments.

"You tell me," I had said. "What do you guys do when the world seems to be bringing you down?"

The responses poured in. Some people said they listened to their favorite music. Others listened to their favorite music *loud*. One woman said she grabbed her kid and went to Disneyland, "the happiest place on earth." One cool chick said she made herself an apple martini, took a bubble bath, watched a movie, and then painted her toes bright red. Some wrote, others exercised, one guy said he behaved like an asshole. I identified with and appreciated something in each response, but one seemed to speak directly to me.

Hi Mia,

My name is M. My daughter and I are fans, and you are very beautiful Sweetie. I'm a grown woman with a daughter your age. I just read your post and have to give you major props for reaching out when you felt the need. Can I try to give you some insight? I have lived a LONG time Mia, and made a ton of mistakes. But, I have been married to my husband for nearly 30 years, and he has multiple sclerosis. I have also faced major major illness of my own. Here's what I have to say, Life is sweet. In between all the bullshit we have to remember something, every moment is a true gift. Of course, we can't live each second in total bliss, that would be impossible. Still, remember to speak to God Sweet Girl. He is there, I promise you. I am no bible thumper, this is what I've discovered. Finding balance in our minds, peace of mind is a priceless endeavor. Sitting with your pet, if you have one. Calling someone you love and connecting. Saying "I love you" after each phone call to those important to you, re-fuels you and also is the catalyst of that becoming the norm. Enjoying a day Mia, just enjoying the moment. It sounds so simple, I know it's not that simple. But, practicing being happy makes you happy. All things that are hard are worthwhile. Having a family that works, takes work. Being content takes work and managing your own life. Remembering arguing and dealing with people that are not good for you and your surroundings is toxic. Going through your relationships in your mind, realizing those that are good for you, and those that are harmful will help you to find balance. Go to the bookstore or library, (me, I dig the library, always have, felt safe there since I was little). Ask someone who works there for a good book. NOT a self-help book, but a great novel, or a funny book. Get lost in it, forget about life for an hour or so and read. It is fertilizer for good thoughts. Replace negative thoughts with positive thoughts. It takes work, but it DOES work. Me, I always use my kids running down the hallway on Christmas morning

*asking, "did Santa come last night?" Think of videos of
yourself younger, and put one of those happy pictures into
your brain and call on it when you need a smile. Remember
to smile, a lot. Even when you feel like crawling inside of
yourself, greeting another with a smile sends out great karma.
Karma comes back to us like boomerangs, might as well make
it as good as we can. Most of all, know that you are good, and
kind, and want the best that life has to offer. Be sweet, go out
of your way to do a good deed. Give yourself kudos for a job
well done. I have to say, you have accomplished much in your
short life, so I know you are capable of anything. I don't know
you personally, I only see you as a Mother would see you. If
you were my daughter I would say I was proud of you Mia. I
would tell you that you make me happy, and that you can do
anything you want to do, including finding a center. There is
nothing like peace of mind. Work to find it. But don't torture
yourself. Man, I've gone on and on, but please know that I
am sincere. I live in New York and you know how crazed it
can be. Yet I love New Yorkers. They will tell you how it is,
and that's what I'm trying to do I suppose. God Bless you
Sweetie, and know that you are NOT alone, we all have to
deal with ourselves daily.*

Peace Honey, M.

In July, I flew to Chicago for a friend's wedding and met a guy who
I dated afterward. I was trying to move on with my life. That's
what I told myself. That's what I told my girlfriends when I reported the facts about the new guy to them. But it was like being
in a meeting and wishing I were someplace else. No matter what
was going on, I kept thinking about Brian.

In early August, I came up to my next tattoo appointment. I
was in the midst of getting a tree on my arm, a tree that had been
partially inspired by one of Brian's tattoos. Prior to our breakup,
he had said that he'd go with me. The appointments took a long

time and I'd liked the idea of having him keep me company. I still liked the idea. I liked it even more than before. I missed him. I wanted to talk to him.

Mustering my courage, I sent him a text, asking if he still planned on going with me.

"No. Sorry. Can't make it," he replied. "Got a job interview."

During my appointment, I found out that he had lied, that there wasn't a job interview. From what I learned, he felt as if he'd made overtures to get back together, but I'd turned him down . . . and yadda-yadda-yadda. It was stupid. On my way back home from the appointment, I called him and said that I wanted to see him.

"Why?" he asked.

I stuttered and stammered and tried to figure out the best— no, the safest response, when I basically thought to myself, *What the fuck are you doing? Just say what's in your heart. Tell him the truth and see what happens.*

"I want to see you because I'm still in love with you."

"But you're with another guy," he said. "Why are you with him? What are you doing to me? Why are you calling me?"

"Shut up," I said. "I'm calling because I am in love with *you*."

We saw each other a handful of times over the next week. There were awkward moments as well as wonderful, loving, memorable moments as each of us tried to figure out where the other stood. I want to say we were grappling with the issue of trust, but looking back I think the real issue was fear—fear of opening our hearts, fear of taking the next step, fear of not knowing if what would happen next was right.

At the end of the month, we decided to go to San Francisco to see a band, and while we were there and I watched him interact and tell stories with his family, I knew that my heart and instincts had been right, and that he was the one. A change also came over him. I could tell that he'd let go of whatever resistance had prevented him from committing before. He dropped his guard. One night I remarked on his love feeling different.

"How so?" he said.

"I don't know. It's like you're vulnerable," I said. "Real."

A few nights later we were in bed. Brian was lying over me, looking in my eyes, and he said, "I want to marry you."

"What?"

"I want to spend the rest of my life with you," he continued. "You're the one. Everything I've gone through in my life has led to you."

I felt the same way—and more, I felt truly blessed. I'd connected with someone who loved me as much as I loved him, and as he'd said, I didn't think any of it would have happened if I hadn't gone through everything that had come before. Things weren't perfect for me. I'd basically raised myself. It sucked that I'd hated my mom. It sucked that my dad hadn't been around as much as I would've liked. It sucked that I had hurt so badly at times that I'd cut myself. It sucked that I'd gotten divorced. But I'd learned from my mistakes. They'd made me stronger.

They'd led to this moment where I hugged Brian so tight that I felt his heart beat against mine. For all the music I'd heard in my life, there was no better sound than the beating of our hearts in love. It made me think. Yeah, I'd gone through some messed-up stuff. But I'd let it go. In turn, I'd created something that I really liked, that made me proud. I'd created myself.

You can do the same thing.

Be patient and tough.
One day this pain will be worth it.

Life isn't about finding yourself.
It's about creating yourself.

Good looking out.

Acknowledgments

Many thanks to my manager, Andrew Lear, Howard Lapides, and everybody at The Core, Sandy Fox at Fox Law Group, and thanks to Dan Strone from Trident Media Group. Without you guys, this book would still just be a bunch of memories in my head.

And a thousand thank-yous to Todd Gold. You have a way with words that is pure magic. You forced me to step outside myself and create something I never thought could be so amazing. You have helped me in more ways than you know, and for that I am forever grateful.

Thanks to all my girls, Gillian, Jennifer, Leah, Courtney, and Angela. Thank you for all that you are. I am so blessed to have you all in my life. It has been a fun ride with you guys so far and I couldn't ask for a better group of friends.

Thanks to my family, Julia, Dad, Chelsea, Taj, Liv, Linda, Laura, and all the rest of the Tallarico clan. This has been an amazing journey so far. I am proud to be a part of such a talented, beautiful, caring family. I love you all so much.

Thank you to Brian. I have finally found you. My great love. I can't wait to get started on our next journey together and be husband and wife . . . to make our own family . . . and do it right! I love you.

And thank you to my mom, Cyrinda. There are no words to say how thankful I am to you. I will never regret any of the choices I have made in my life because those are the things that have made me who I am today. My only regret is that you are not here to share in my joys and sorrows anymore. No one will understand the love I have for you. It grows stronger with every day. But that is between us. I know I don't say it enough, but I love you.